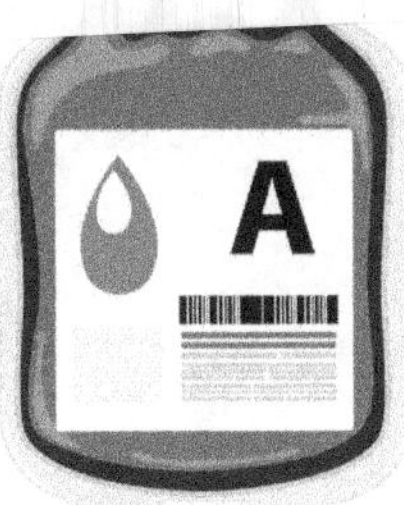

Eat Well

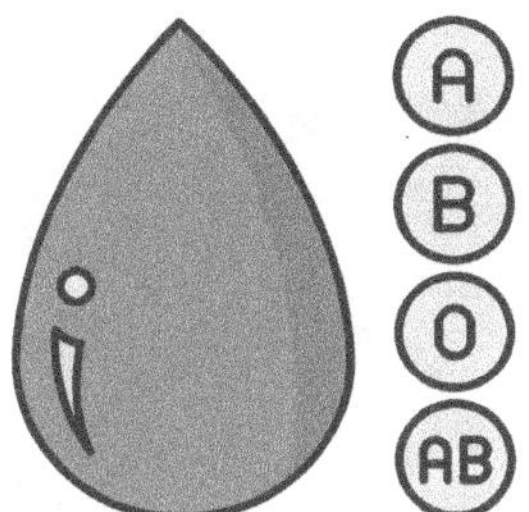

4

Your Blood Type

A Customized Cookbook with Over 150 Nourishing Recipes for Type A Dieters

Sarah William & Dr. Vivian Greene

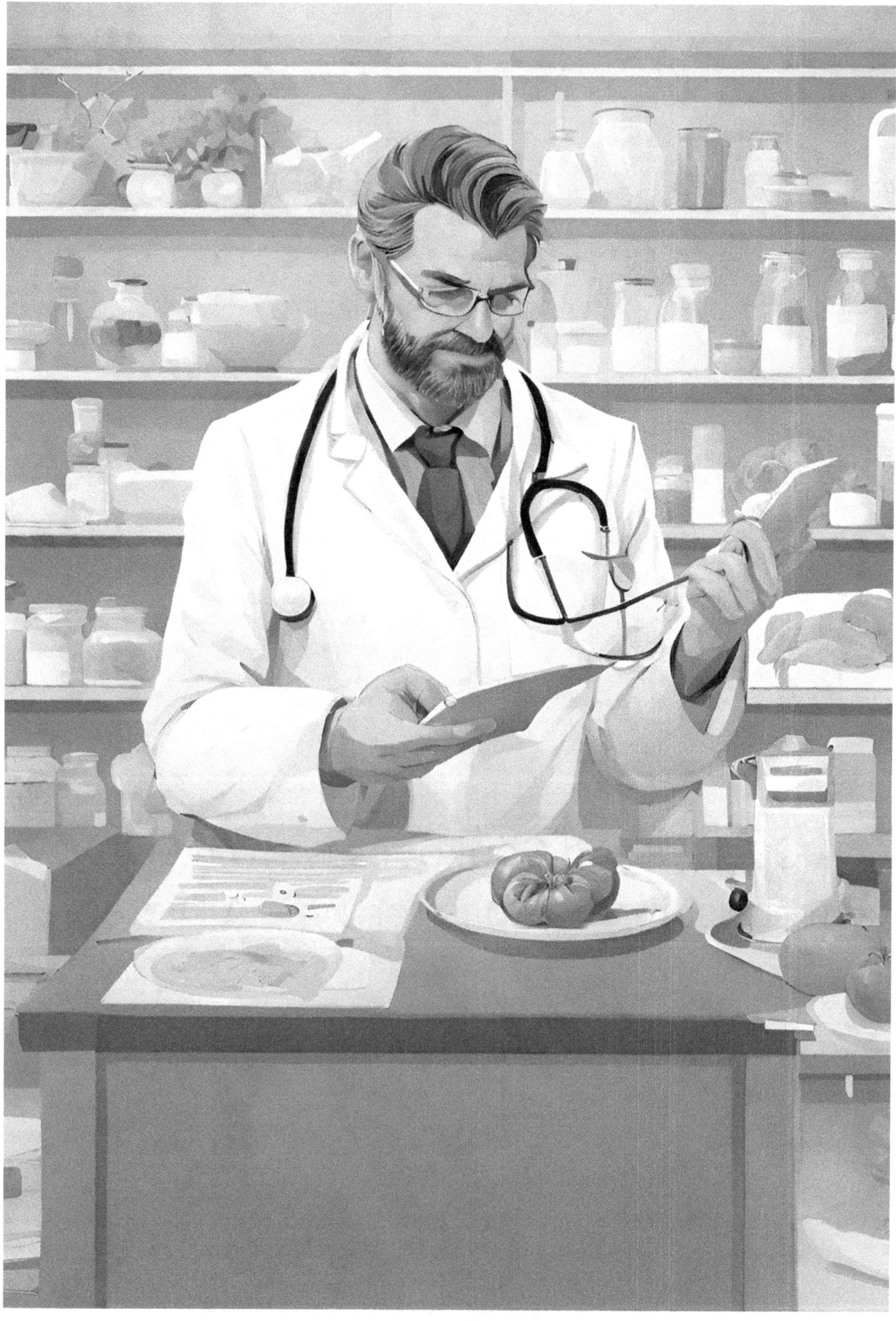

Copyright © 2024 by Sarah William & Dr. Vivian Greene

Disclaimer

The information provided in this cookbook is for educational and informational purposes only and is not intended as medical advice. Consult with a qualified healthcare professional before making any dietary or lifestyle changes, especially if you have any underlying health conditions or concerns. The authors, Sarah William & Dr. Vivian Greene, and the publisher disclaim any liability for any adverse effects or consequences resulting from the use of the information provided in this cookbook. The reader assumes full responsibility for their actions and decisions based on the information contained herein.

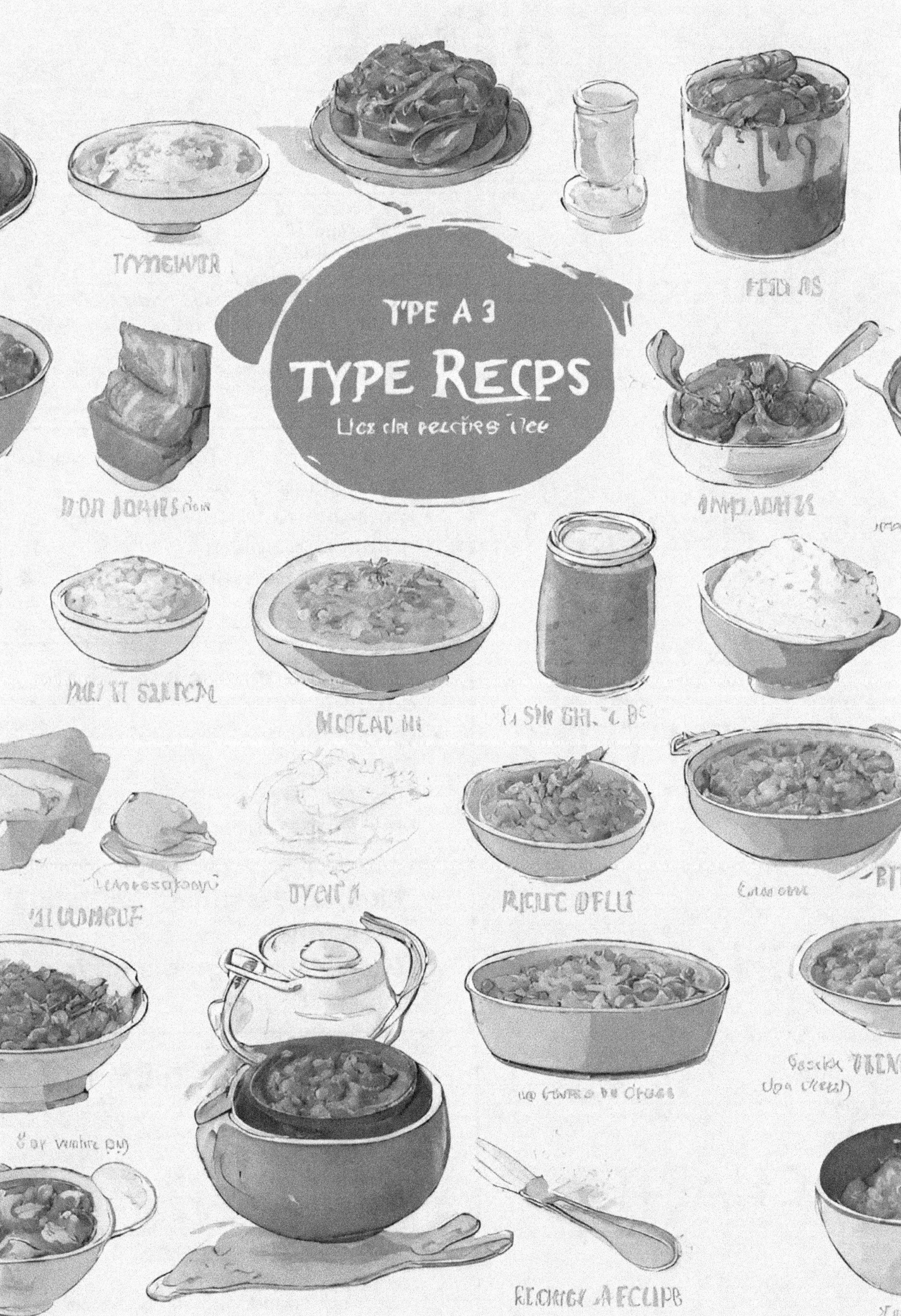
TYPE RECPS

TABLE
Of Contents

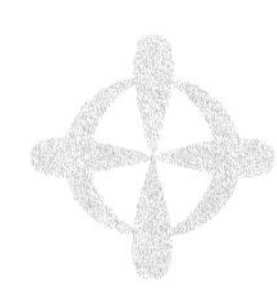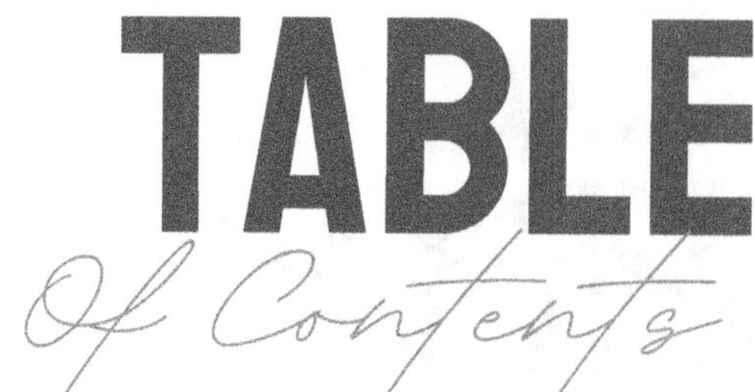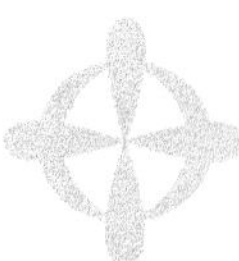

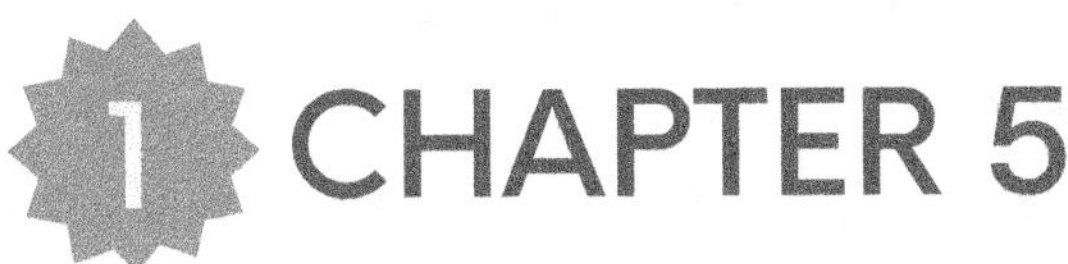

CHAPTER 5

Lunch Recipes

- Quinoa Salad with Chickpeas and Vegetables
- Lentil and Vegetable Soup
- Tofu Stir-Fry with Broccoli and Bell Peppers
- Chickpea and Avocado Wrap
- Mediterranean Quinoa Bowl
- Spinach and Strawberry Salad with Balsamic Vinaigrette
- Veggie and Hummus Wrap
- Greek Lentil Salad
- Veggie and Tofu Stir-Fry with Brown Rice
- Mediterranean Chickpea Salad

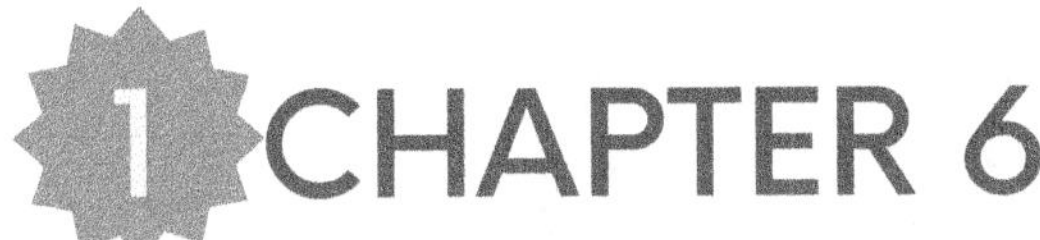

CHAPTER 6

Dinner Recipes

- Quinoa-Stuffed Bell Peppers
- Lemon Herb Baked Salmon
- Mediterranean Chickpea Salad
- Vegetable Stir-Fry with Tofu
- Lentil and Vegetable Curry
- Grilled Vegetable Skewers
- Eggplant and Chickpea Tagine
- Spinach and Mushroom Quiche
- Turkey and Vegetable Lettuce Wraps
- Vegetable and Tofu Stir-Fry with Brown Rice

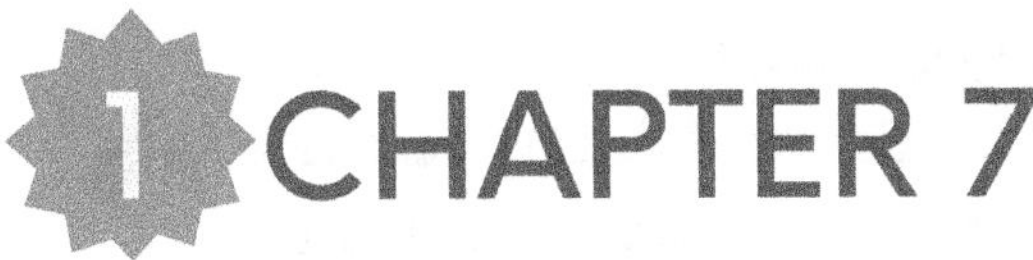

CHAPTER 7

Snack Recipes

- Avocado Toast with Tomato and Basil
- Greek Yogurt with Berries and Almonds
- Hummus and Veggie Sticks
- Almond Butter Banana Slices
- Quinoa Salad Cups
- Rice Cake with Almond Butter and Banana
- Edamame Salad
- Cottage Cheese with Pineapple
- Stuffed Bell Pepper Halves
- Apple Slices with Almond Butter and Chia Seeds

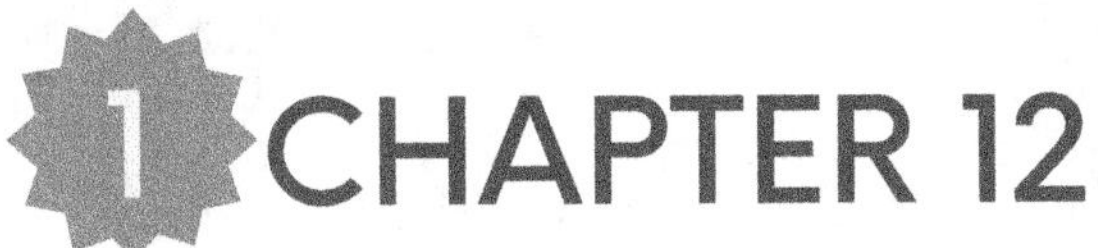

CHAPTER 12

- **Frequently Asked Questions (FAQs)**
- **Conclusion**

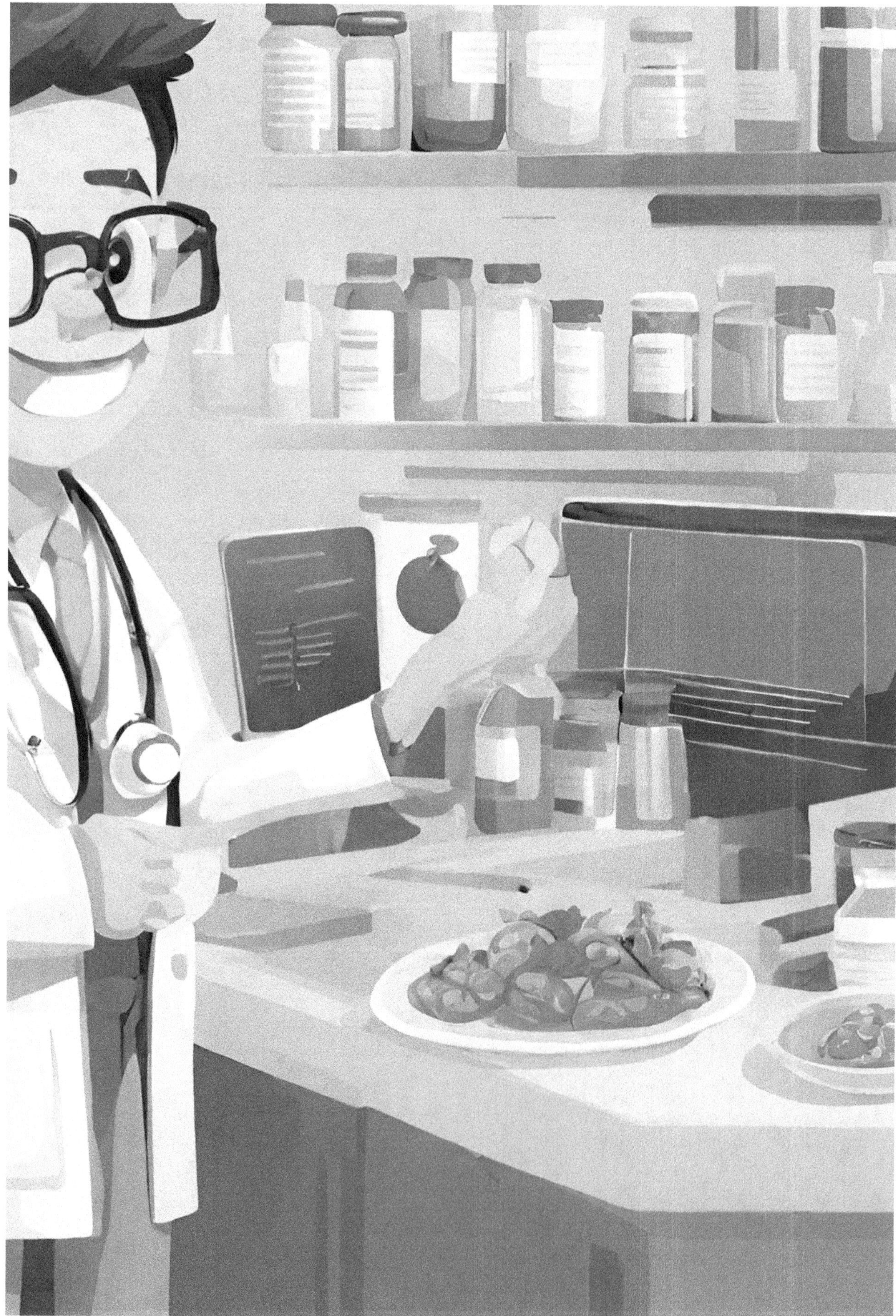

Introduction

Welcome to "Eat Well for Your Blood Type: A Customized Cookbook," a revolutionary cookbook designed to transform your perspective on health and nutrition. This book, written by eminent medical experts and supported by the most recent scientific findings, offers a customized nutrition plan made especially for people with Type A blood.

We sympathize with those who are frustrated by the abundance of one-size-fits-all diet plans and generic diet plans available on the market and would like a more customized approach to nutrition. For this reason, we have thoroughly investigated the complex connection between blood type and nutritional needs to provide you with a thorough resource that goes beyond the accepted guidelines for a balanced diet.
With decades of combined experience in holistic wellness, medicine, and nutrition, our team of highly qualified experts has carefully selected more than 150 nutritious meals to help support and enhance the health of Type A dieters. However, this cookbook is more than simply a list of mouthwatering recipes; it's also evidence of the effectiveness of customized nutrition in reaching robust health and energy.

Along the way, you'll learn the special advantages of Type A personalities, the science behind blood type diets, and useful advice for incorporating these ideas into your everyday life. Regardless of your level of experience in the kitchen, our approachable style guarantees that you'll find motivation and direction at every step.

However, there is a deeper philosophy that goes beyond cookbooks and meal plans—one that acknowledges the significant influence that food has on our mental, emotional, and spiritual health. By following the advice in "Eat Well for Your Blood Type," you're not only providing your body with nourishment, but you're also respecting its particular requirements and opening the door to a lifetime of ideal health.

So come along for the ride as we go on a gastronomic adventure catered to your Type A blood type. Allow this cookbook to serve as your dependable guide, your health's lighthouse, and the opening to a happier, more energetic future.

The Concept of Eating According to Your Blood Type

The idea behind eating for your blood type is the theory that each person has different dietary needs depending on their blood type. Numerous publications and studies that proposed a link between blood type and dietary requirements helped popularize this theory.

This theory's proponents contend that blood type affects how our bodies absorb and digest certain meals as well as how our immune systems react to various food ingredients. This idea states that following a blood-type-specific diet may help control weight, improve digestion, optimize health, and increase energy levels.

Blood type diet proponents, for example, contend that those with Type A blood may benefit from a diet high in fruits, vegetables, legumes, and whole grains that are predominantly plant-based. This is allegedly because people with Type A blood are thought to have sensitive immune systems and might benefit from a diet heavy in complex carbohydrates and low in animal proteins.

On the other hand, those with Type O blood are sometimes recommended to eat like that of prehistoric hunter-gatherer tribes, which emphasize fruits, vegetables, and animal proteins while avoiding grains and dairy. This is predicated on the idea that people with Type O blood could have stronger digestive systems and would do better on a diet heavier in protein and lower in carbohydrates.

Although the idea of eating according to your blood type has been met with both enthusiasm and skepticism in the scientific world, there isn't much hard data to back it up. Although certain studies have hinted at possible links between blood type and particular health outcomes, a more thorough investigation is required to support these theories.

Irrespective of its scientific validity, many people who are looking for a customized approach to nutrition find resonance in the concept of adjusting dietary choices to individual requirements. Whether you decide to follow the blood type diet or not, respecting your body's individual needs is always essential to overall health and well-being.

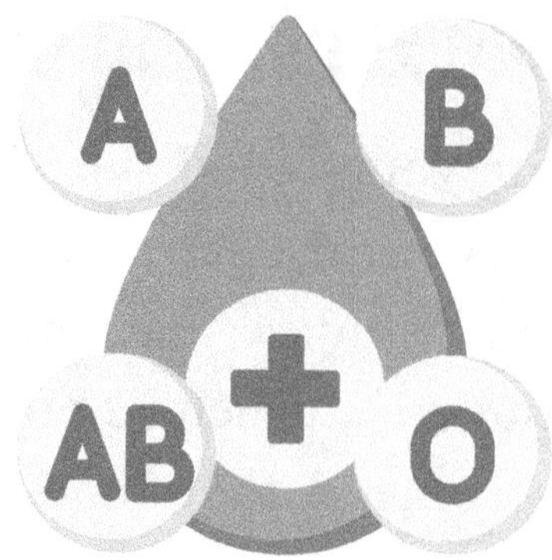

Understanding Your Blood Type

Knowing your blood type is essential to following the blood type diet and related dietary guidelines. Type A, Type B, Type AB, and Type O are the four primary blood types. Specific antigens on the surface of red blood cells and the presence or lack of antibodies in plasma identify each blood type.

Type A: Red blood cells with A antigens and plasma with anti-B antibodies are characteristics of people with Type A blood. This blood type is said to have come from agrarian communities and is linked to characteristics like sensitivity, inventiveness, and adaptability. Type A people are often advised to have a mostly plant-based diet that is high in fruits, vegetables, legumes, and whole grains within the framework of the blood type diet.

Type B: Plasma contains anti-A antibodies and red blood cells with B antigens. It is believed that this blood type originated in people who were nomadic and is linked to traits like resilience, flexibility, and adaptability. An eclectic diet that balances meats, dairy, grains, fruits, and vegetables may be advantageous for those with Type B blood.

Type AB blood has red blood cells that have both A and B antigens on them, as well as a low level of anti-A and anti-B antibodies in the plasma. This blood type is thought to be somewhat uncommon and is linked to characteristics like complexity, inventiveness, and adaptability. People with Type AB blood may benefit from a diet that incorporates foods from several food categories and components of Type A and Type B guidelines.

Type O: The plasma of type O blood has both anti-A and anti-B antibodies, but the red blood cells lack the A and B antigens. Known as the "universal donor," this blood type is said to have come from early hunter-gatherer cultures. Generally speaking, type O people are recommended to restrict grains and dairy products and have a diet high in fruits, vegetables, and animal proteins.

Knowing your blood type might provide you with important information about possible food sensitivity and preferences. Although blood type diets are still controversial among medical experts, many people find that eating a diet according to their blood type helps enhance their general health, energy, and digestion. Any dietary adjustments, nevertheless, must be done carefully and after consulting a healthcare professional.

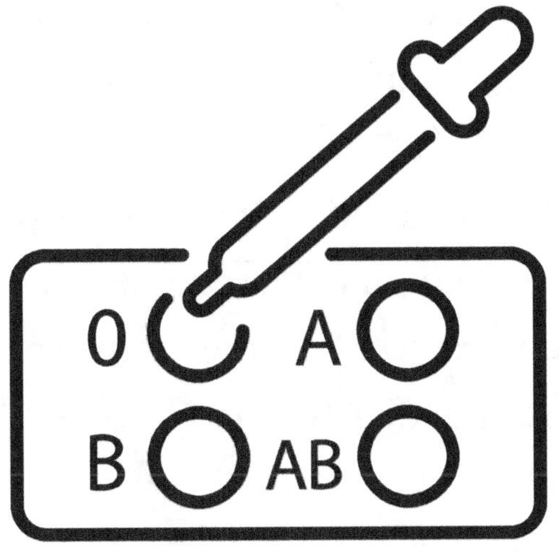

Characteristics of Type A Blood

Type A blood has more traits than only physical qualities; it also involves behavioral inclinations, vulnerability to certain medical diseases, and perhaps food preferences. The following are some essential traits that people with Type A blood are often known for:

Adaptability: People with Type A blood are often said to be sensitive to environmental changes and adaptable. They could have an acute sense of awareness of their surroundings and do better in environments that are well-organized and structured.

Sensitivity: People who are type A tend to be very perceptive and empathic, with a profound comprehension of the feelings and viewpoints of others. They could place a higher value on harmony and collaboration in their interactions and relationships.

Creativity: It is believed that people with Type A blood have a penchant for the creative and artistic. Using their creativity and expressiveness, they might be excellent in creative endeavors like writing, music, or the visual arts.

Stress Reaction: Compared to other blood types, type A personalities are believed to have a more sensitive stress reaction. Effective stress management techniques are necessary since people are more likely to experience elevated levels of stress and anxiety under challenging circumstances.

Digestive Sensitivity: Some blood type diet proponents speculate that Type A personalities may have more sensitive digestive systems, especially when it comes to how they absorb certain foods. They could thus benefit from a diet that emphasizes foods that are easily digested and plant-based.

Susceptibility to Specific Health Conditions: Blood type does not by itself indicate a person's health status, although some research indicates that people with Type A blood may be more vulnerable to specific illnesses, including cancer and heart disease. To prove a definitive connection, further research is necessary.

It is crucial to remember that these traits are based on broad generalizations and could not apply to every person with Type A blood. A person's personality characteristics and health outcomes may also be greatly influenced by lifestyle decisions, environmental influences, and individual variances.

Gaining knowledge about the traits linked to Type A blood may be quite beneficial in terms of identifying possible advantages, weaknesses, and nutritional needs. To fully appreciate the intricate web of interrelated elements that shape each person's own identity and well-being, it is essential to approach these interpretations with an open mind and a critical eye.

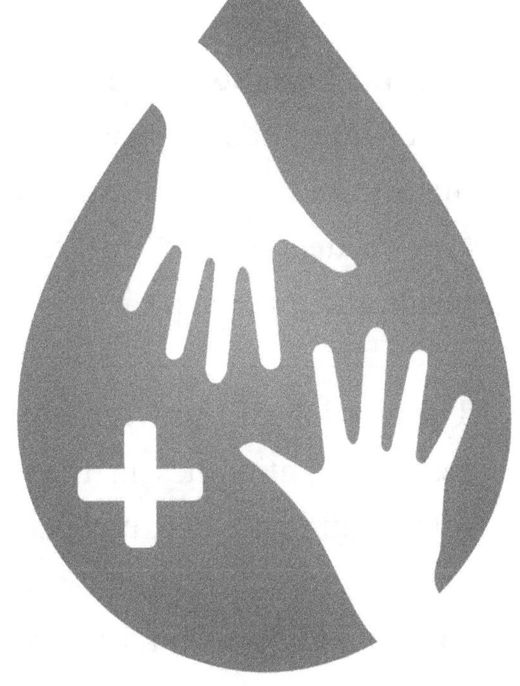

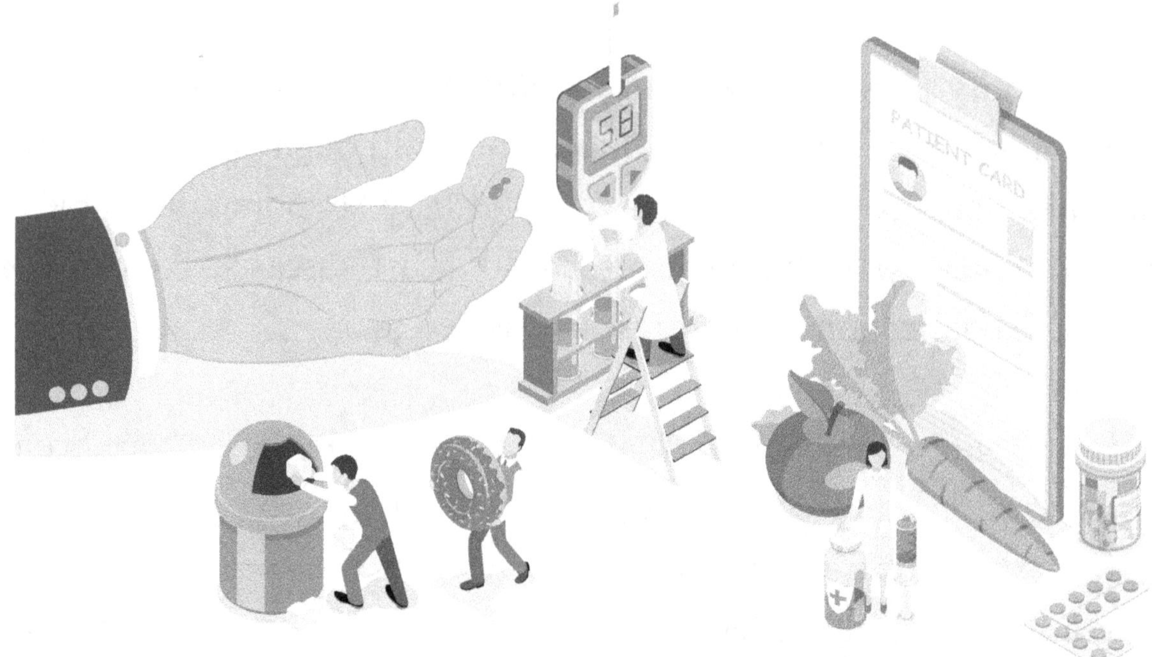

The Science Behind Blood Type Diets

Within the fields of nutrition and medical research, there is continuous investigation and discussion on the science behind blood-type diets. Blood type diet proponents contend that a person's blood type affects how their body reacts to certain meals and nutrients, which may affect general health and well-being. Blood type diets are justified by numerous important considerations, even if the idea is still debatable:

Genetic Variation: The foundation of blood type diets is the idea that over thousands of years, various blood types formed in response to dietary and environmental stimuli. Proponents hypothesize that blood type-related genetic differences may affect how people digest certain meals and minerals.

The relationship between blood-type antigens on the surface of red blood cells and antibodies in the circulation is a topic that blood-type diets often highlight. Because people with Type A blood, for instance, have anti-B antibodies, supporters advise against eating specific foods that contain antigens that are incompatible with their blood type.

Inflammatory Responses: Some blood type diet proponents contend that some foods may cause inflammatory reactions in people of particular blood types, which may exacerbate long-term medical concerns. It has been suggested that people may enhance their general health and minimize inflammation by customizing their diet to match their blood type.

Nutrient Absorption and Digestion: Another theory supporting blood type diets is that blood types may affect an individual's capacity to efficiently absorb and digest certain nutrients. Proponents speculate, for example, that those with Type O blood could be more tolerant of animal proteins, while people with Type A blood might do better on a diet heavy in plants.

Personalized Nutrition: The fundamental idea behind blood type diets is to promote customized eating according to each person's unique physiological makeup. Proponents contend that people may optimize nutritional intake, enhance metabolic health, and lower their chance of developing certain medical diseases by matching their dietary choices to their blood type.

Blood type diets are still supported by a small and conflicting body of scientific research, despite some observational studies suggesting possible links between blood type and certain health outcomes. The theories supporting blood type diets, according to critics, are not well supported by science and may oversimplify the intricate interactions between genetic, environmental, and lifestyle variables that affect dietary needs and health consequences.

although there are still discussion and study around the effectiveness of blood-type diets in promoting health and avoiding illness. While some people may benefit from adhering to a blood-type diet, others could gain more from taking a more evidence-based, balanced approach to nutrition that takes into account eating habits, personal preferences, and overall health objectives.

Origins and Development of Blood Type Diets

Blood type diets may be traced back to the work of two naturopathic physicians, Dr. Peter D'Adamo and his father, James D'Adamo, who was also a naturopath. Dr. Peter D'Adamo postulated in the late 20th century that a person's blood type may have an impact on their nutritional requirements and general health.

Dr. D'Adamo's observations of his patients' reactions to various diets according to their blood types gave rise to the idea. According to his theory, people's blood types may determine which foods are more or less healthy for them, and adjusting one's diet appropriately might result in better health.

After Dr. D'Adamo's book "Eat Right for Your Type" was published in 1996, his views became well known. He suggested that following the dietary recommendations for each blood type—Type O, Type A, Type B, and Type AB—could improve energy levels, promote optimal health, and lower the chance of developing several diseases.

Blood type diets saw a sharp increase in popularity, drawing defenders who spoke of their success as well as detractors who questioned the concept's scientific foundation. Regardless of the debate, blood type diets remained popular due to testimonies, celebrity endorsements, and the abundance of publications, websites, and merchandise endorsing the strategy.

The original blood type diet underwent many revisions and alterations throughout time, with various writers and proponents contributing their analyses and changes. Some proponents broadened the notion to include lifestyle elements other than nutrition, such as suggested exercise regimens and stress-reduction strategies.

Blood type diets have their roots in the research of Dr. Peter D'Adamo, but it's vital to remember that many people and organizations have modified and expanded on the idea throughout time. Blood type diets are still a subject of discussion and interest in the domains of nutrition, alternative medicine, and holistic health today. While supporters of the practice urge prudence and further research, detractors urge caution.

Scientific Basis and Research Supporting Blood Type Diets

In the scientific community, there has been much discussion and examination of the data and scientific foundations supporting blood type diets. Blood type diet proponents believe that their individualized approach to nutrition is based on blood type, while their detractors argue that the evidence for their effectiveness is weak and ambiguous.

Blood type diet proponents assert that the idea is based on several scientific grounds, such as:

Genetic Variability: Blood type diets are based on the idea that people vary genetically from one another, and that this affects how their bodies react to various meals. Blood type antigens and antibodies, among other hereditary characteristics, are said to have an impact on immune system performance, nutrition, metabolism, and general health.

Blood type diets place a strong emphasis on the relationship between blood type antigens on red blood cells and antibodies in the blood. Because people with Type A blood have anti-B antibodies, supporters advise against eating specific foods that contain antigens that are incompatible with their blood type to avoid negative responses.

According to some advocates, eating certain foods may cause inflammatory reactions in people with particular blood types, which may aggravate long-term medical concerns including inflammation, autoimmune illnesses, and metabolic abnormalities. People may allegedly lessen inflammation and improve general health by matching their food choices to their blood type.

Blood type diets posit that an individual's blood type may have an impact on their capacity to efficiently absorb and digest certain nutrients. Proponents speculate, for example, that those with Type O blood could be more tolerant of animal proteins, while people with Type A blood might do better on a diet heavy in plants.

Although these ideas seem reasonable at first glance, there is still a paucity of contradictory scientific data to back up blood type diets. Critics say that many of the ideas behind blood type diets are not backed up by strong scientific evidence and may oversimplify the complex ways that genetic, environmental, and lifestyle factors interact to determine dietary needs and health outcomes.

Numerous research endeavors have endeavored to explore the plausible correlations between blood type and diverse health consequences, such as susceptibility to illnesses, nutritional processing, and dietary choices. Nevertheless, the findings have been mixed, with some research pointing to weak associations and others finding no meaningful connection.

Regarding the effectiveness and validity of blood type diets, the scientific community is still split overall. Although some people may claim to have subjective advantages from adhering to a blood type diet, it is crucial to approach such dietary suggestions with care and skepticism since there is a dearth of solid scientific data to support their efficiency. To clarify the possible processes underpinning blood type diets and their effects on health outcomes, further study is required.

CHAPTER 1

Benefits of Eating According to Your Blood Type

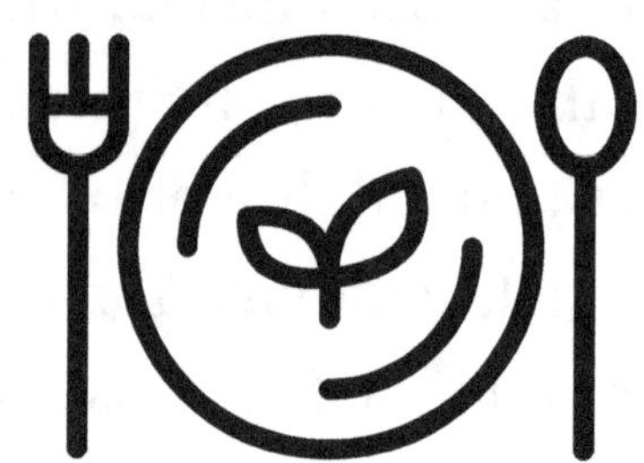

Blood type diet proponents have discussed and shown interest in the potential advantages of eating based on your blood type. Although there is ongoing discussion on the scientific veracity of these claims, supporters point to several possible advantages of matching one's food choices to one's blood type:

tailored Nutrition: The blood type diet's focus on tailored nutrition is one of its main points of support. Proponents hypothesize that due to hereditary variables such as blood type antigens and antibodies, people with various blood types may have particular dietary requirements and tolerances. People may enhance their general health and well-being and maximize their nutritional intake by customizing their diets to match their blood type.

Better Digestion: Blood type diet proponents contend that depending on an individual's blood type, certain foods may be easier for them to digest and absorb. People may lessen their chance of experiencing bloating, digestive pain, and other gastrointestinal problems by avoiding foods that are thought to be incompatible with their blood type. This may enhance digestive health and general well-being.

Weight control: According to some blood type diet proponents, matching one's food choices to one's blood type may help with weight control. Although there is no scientific evidence to back this concept, people may enjoy better hunger control, an improved metabolism, and superior weight loss results by concentrating on foods that are supposedly favorable for their blood type and avoiding those that are not.

Enhanced Vitality: Blood-type diet proponents often cite heightened vitality and energy levels as possible advantages of adhering to a blood-type-specific diet. People who eat foods thought to be suitable for their blood type may feel less tired, have more concentration and mental clarity, and have maintained energy throughout the day.

Decreased Risk of Health Conditions: Although there is no scientific proof to back up this assertion, some advocates contend that eating by your blood type may lower your chance of developing certain illnesses and ailments. For instance, those with Type A blood are often recommended to eat a diet high in plant-based foods, since this may help reduce the risk of obesity, heart disease, and several types of cancer. To confirm these correlations and pinpoint the precise role that blood type diets play in disease prevention, further investigation is necessary.

All things considered, the supposed advantages of eating by your blood type highlight the significance of customized nutrition and the possible impact of hereditary variables on dietary needs and health results. Individual experiences may differ, but given the paucity of solid scientific data proving blood-type diets effective, it's imperative to examine such dietary advice critically and skeptically.

Personalized Nutrition and Its Impact on Health

Personalized nutrition refers to a comprehensive approach to food and lifestyle that customizes nutritional guidelines and treatments based on individual traits such as genetic composition, metabolic profile, state of health, and personal preferences. Personalized nutrition strives to maximize health outcomes, avoid illness, and enhance general well-being by taking these variables into account. Personalized nutrition may have the following effects on health:

Optimum nutritional consumption: Individual nutritional needs are considered via personalized nutrition, which takes into consideration variables like age, gender, degree of exercise, and health. Personalized nutrition programs may make sure people are getting enough of the vital vitamins, minerals, and nutrients they need to perform at their best by evaluating these variables.

Better Digestive Health: An individualized diet may help reduce digestive problems including gas, indigestion, bloating, and constipation by choosing meals that are readily digested and well-tolerated for each individual. A person's gut health and optimal nutrient absorption may be enhanced by customizing their diet to suit their unique digestive requirements.

Optimized Weight Control: By addressing the unique elements that influence weight gain or reduction, personalized nutrition plans may help achieve weight management objectives. This might include taking into account elements like dietary preferences, lifestyle choices, hormonal balance, and metabolic rate while creating a nutrition plan. Personalized nutrition may help with long-term weight reduction or maintenance by tailoring dietary advice to each person's requirements.

The prevention and management of illnesses: By targeting underlying risk factors and encouraging healthy lifestyle habits, personalized nutrition has the potential to lower the risk of chronic diseases including cancer, diabetes, heart disease, and metabolic syndrome.

Dietary therapies targeting the reduction of cholesterol and enhancement of cardiovascular health may be advantageous for those with a familial history of heart disease.

Increased Vitality and Energy Levels: A tailored diet may boost vitality and energy levels while lowering weariness and giving the body the resources it needs to perform at its best. Well-proportioned meals that are customized to meet specific dietary needs may help maintain energy levels all day, encourage physical activity, and improve concentration and mental clarity.

Optimal athletic performance may be achieved through personalized nutrition, which gives athletes the proper ratio of macronutrients (proteins, fats, and carbs) and micronutrients (vitamins and minerals) to support their training, recuperation, and performance objectives. Personalized nutrition may improve endurance, strength, and general athletic performance by tailoring meal regimens to the unique requirements of athletes.

All things considered, customized nutrition provides a diet and lifestyle strategy that takes into account unique traits and requirements. Personalized nutrition may significantly influence general health and well-being by improving nutrient intake, fostering digestive health, aiding in weight control, avoiding illness, and boosting vitality and energy levels.

Specific Benefits for Type A Dieters

Blood type diet proponents assert that type A dieters may benefit more specifically from a diet that is customized for their blood type. Although these assertions are controversial and need further research to be confirmed, supporters list several possible benefits for those with Type A blood:

Better Digestive Health: Dieters who follow the type A protocol are often recommended to eat a diet high in fruits, vegetables, legumes, and whole grains that are predominantly plant-based. Foods that are thought to be compatible with the digestive tract of people with Type A blood may lower the risk of gastrointestinal problems such as bloating and pain. Dieters who follow a Type A diet and concentrate on easily digested plant-based meals may see an improvement in their digestive health and regularity.

Decreased chance of chronic diseases: According to some blood type diet proponents, eating a diet that corresponds with one's blood type may reduce the chance of developing chronic conditions, including cancer, obesity, and heart disease. A plant-based diet rich in fruits and vegetables that supports heart health helps Type A dieters maintain a healthy weight, and reduces inflammation may provide preventive effects against these illnesses. Nevertheless, further investigation is required to validate these correlations.

Enhanced Immune Function: Type A personalities' diets, which place a strong focus on nutrient-rich plant foods, may help to strengthen both the immune system and general health. Rich in vitamins, minerals, and antioxidants, fruits and vegetables support a healthy immune system and guard against infections and diseases. Type A dieters may benefit from improved immune function and increased resilience to common diseases by eating a diet high in immune-boosting foods.

Support for Weight Control: Plant-based diets may be helpful for type A dieters in achieving their weight control objectives. Plant-based diets are often lower in calories and saturated fats than animal-based diets, which makes them beneficial for attempts to lose or maintain weight. Furthermore, the high fiber content of plant-based meals might help Type A personalities maintain a healthy weight by increasing fullness and decreasing food cravings.

Enhanced Energy: Type A dieters may have prolonged energy throughout the day due to the nutrient-dense character of a plant-based diet. Whole grains, legumes, and vegetables include complex carbs, which release energy gradually to minimize energy crashes and support stable blood sugar levels. Plant-based diets high in nutrients may help Type A dieters feel more energized, more clear-headed, and more vital all around.

Although supporters of blood type diets for Type A personalities often mention these possible advantages, it's crucial to view such claims with prudence and skepticism. There is still a dearth of solid scientific data proving the effectiveness of blood-type diets, particularly about Type A dieters. Individual results may differ, as with any dietary strategy; thus, speaking with a healthcare provider is advised before making big dietary adjustments based on blood type guidelines.

CHAPTER
2
Getting Started: How to Use This Cookbook

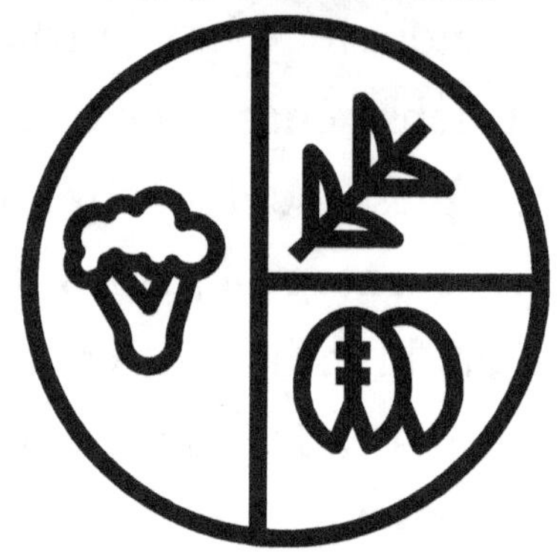

Making the most of a cookbook's contents and savoring the culinary adventure it provides requires adeptly navigating its pages. Here are some pointers on using this cookbook to improve your culinary skills and find delicious dishes catered to your blood type: Type A

Start by reading the cookbook's introductory section, which contains important details on the blood type diet, its tenets, and how the dishes in this book are geared toward Type A dieters. Gaining an understanding of the cookbook's underlying idea will help you understand why certain dishes and ingredients are suggested for your blood type.

Table of Contents: To get an idea of the recipes included in the cookbook, take some time to go over the table of contents. To make it simpler to locate recipes that fit your meal tastes and dietary requirements, the table of contents arranges recipes into categories including breakfast, lunch, supper, snacks, and desserts.

Recipe Selection: Take into account elements like ingredients, cooking methods, and preparation time when choosing which dishes to test.

Examine the titles and descriptions of the recipes to see whether they fit your nutritional needs and taste preferences. To add variation to your meals, search for recipes that suit certain events or make use of seasonal items.

Ingredient Lists and Substitutions: Make sure you have all the ingredients on hand by carefully reading the ingredient list before beginning a recipe. Check the cookbook's recommendations and ideas for substitutes if you're lacking any items or would rather prepare your own. Because of their adaptability, you may alter recipes to fit your nutritional requirements and tastes.

Cooking directions: Carefully follow each recipe's step-by-step cooking directions, paying close attention to specifics such as cooking temperatures, timings, and methods. The purpose of the instructions is to successfully lead you through the cooking procedure and guarantee excellent outcomes. See the cookbook's culinary tips and advice for help if you're not experienced in the kitchen or if you don't know how to do anything.

Nutritional Data: The cookbook has several recipes with comprehensive nutritional data, including serving sizes, macronutrient breakdowns, and calorie counts. Utilize this data to monitor your nutritional consumption and make well-informed choices regarding portion sizes. Additionally, you may use the nutritional information to help you remember your dietary objectives and make any necessary modifications.

Variety and Exploration: Feel free to experiment and try out the many recipes and ingredients that are included in the cookbook. Adding diversity to your meals may guarantee that you get a balanced range of nutrients and make your diet engaging and pleasurable. Feel free to be creative in the kitchen and modify recipes to fit your tastes.

You may confidently and enthusiastically go on a culinary journey catered to your Type A blood type by paying attention to these pointers on how to utilize this cookbook. This cookbook is meant to encourage you to make tasty, nutritious meals that promote your health and well-being, regardless of your level of culinary expertise. Savor the adventure of tasting new foods, broadening your cooking skills, and accepting the idea of customized eating.

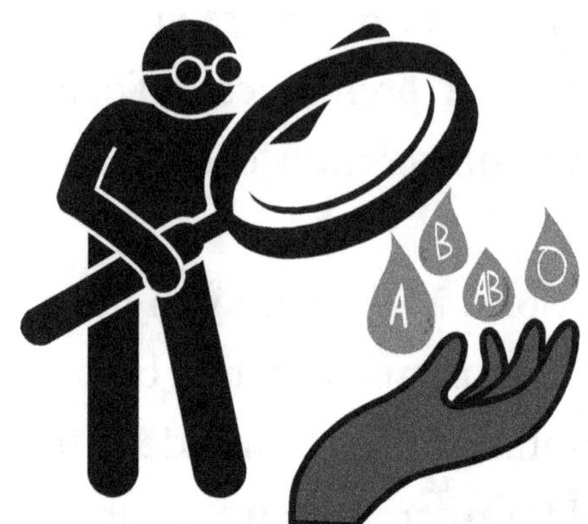

Guidelines for Identifying Your Blood Type

Finding out your blood type is a simple procedure that usually involves having a blood test done by a medical practitioner. However, there are a few other approaches and recommendations you may use to assist in establishing your blood type if you're interested in it and can't get medical testing:

Speak with Your Healthcare Provider: A blood test performed by a medical practitioner is the most dependable and accurate method of determining your blood type. If your blood type is necessary for medical purposes or as part of a normal checkup, your doctor may arrange a blood type test.

Examine Medical Records: Your blood type may be included in your medical records if you've ever had any surgeries or blood transfusions. To get this information, you may ask your healthcare practitioner or medical institution for access to your medical records.

Blood Donation facilities: As part of the donation procedure, blood type is often done in blood donation facilities. If you have already given blood, you may be able to find out your blood type by getting in touch with the blood donation facility where you gave your blood.

Family History: Since blood types are inherited from parents, you may be able to determine your blood type by comparing the blood types of your siblings or biological parents. Because blood type inheritance may be more complicated than a straightforward ABO blood type chart, this approach is not always correct.

Blood Typing Kits: Over-the-counter blood typing kits are available that claim to be able to identify your blood type from a finger prick blood sample. Although these kits may tell you some information about your blood type, you should take care when using them since they might not be as accurate as laboratory testing.

Observation of Blood Features: Although not proven, some people think that certain physical attributes or features could be connected to particular blood types. For instance, people with Type O blood are commonly said to be "universal donors," while those with Type A blood can be more vulnerable to certain diseases. These correlations have not been verified by science and are just anecdotal.

It's crucial to remember that while these techniques could reveal your blood type in part, they are not as accurate as laboratory testing carried out by a medical practitioner. See your doctor or other healthcare practitioner for advice if you're not sure of your blood type or need precise information for medical reasons.

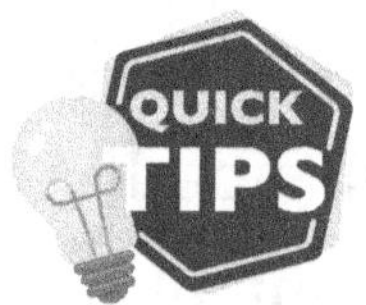

Tips for Grocery Shopping and Meal Preparation

Grocery shopping and meal preparation are essential aspects of maintaining a healthy diet tailored to your blood type. Here are some tips for efficient grocery shopping and meal preparation, along with a list of blood type A-friendly foods to include in your shopping list:

Tips for Grocery Shopping and Meal Preparation:

1.**Plan Ahead:** Before heading to the grocery store, take some time to plan your meals for the week. Consider your schedule, dietary preferences, and any special occasions that may influence your meal choices.

2.**Make a List:** Create a grocery list based on your meal plan to ensure you have all the ingredients you need. Organize your list by food categories (e.g., fruits, vegetables, proteins) to streamline your shopping trip.

3.**Stick to the Perimeter:** Focus on shopping for fresh, whole foods located around the perimeter of the grocery store, such as fruits, vegetables, lean proteins, and dairy products. These items are typically less processed and more nutrient-dense.

4.**Read Labels:** When selecting packaged foods, read the nutrition labels carefully to identify any ingredients that may not be suitable for your blood type. Look for minimally processed, whole-food options with simple ingredient lists.

5.**Choose Seasonal Produce:** Opt for seasonal fruits and vegetables whenever possible, as they tend to be fresher, more flavorful, and more affordable. Seasonal produce also offers variety and supports local agriculture.

6.Buy in Bulk: Consider purchasing staple items such as grains, legumes, nuts, and seeds in bulk to save money and reduce packaging waste. Store bulk items in airtight containers to maintain freshness.

7.Stock Up on Essentials: Keep your pantry stocked with essential ingredients for quick and easy meal preparation, such as whole grains, canned beans, olive oil, herbs, and spices. Having these items on hand ensures you can whip up a nutritious meal anytime.

8.Meal Prep: Dedicate some time each week to meal prep, such as washing and chopping fruits and vegetables, cooking grains and proteins, and portioning out snacks. This will save time during busy weekdays and help you make healthier choices.

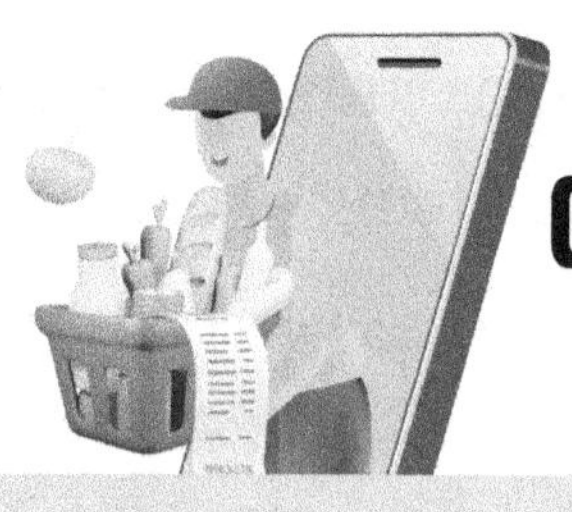

Grocery Shopping List for Blood Type A Dieters

Fruits:	Vegetables:	Proteins:	Whole Grains:	Healthy Fats
Apples	Spinach	Tofu	Quinoa	Avocado
Berries	Kale	Tempeh	Brown rice	Olive oil
(blueberries,	Broccoli	Lentils	Buckwheat	Coconut oil
strawberries,	Brussels	Chickpeas	Oats	Flaxseed oil
raspberries)	sprouts	Black beans	Barley	
Cherries	Cauliflower	Edamame	Millet	
Grapes	Carrots	Eggs	Amaranth	
Pineapple	Sweet	Skinless		
Papaya	potatoes	poultry		
Plums	Bell peppers	(chicken,		
Mango	Cucumber	turkey)		
Kiwi	Zucchini	Wild-caught		
Watermelon		fish (salmon,		
		trout)		

Herbs and Spices

Basil
Parsley
Cilantro
Garlic
Ginger
Turmeric
Cinnamon
Cumin
Paprika

Dairy and Alternatives

Greek yogurt (plain, low-fat)
Almond milk
Soy milk
Goat cheese
Feta cheese

Miscellaneous

Honey
Maple syrup
Dark chocolate (70% cocoa or higher)
Herbal teas
Whole grain bread or wraps

Nuts and Seeds

Almonds
Walnuts
Flaxseeds
Chia seeds
Pumpkin seeds
Sunflower seeds

Remember to adapt this list based on your individual preferences, dietary restrictions, and meal plan. With careful planning and mindful shopping, you can create delicious and nourishing meals tailored to your blood type A diet.

CHAPTER 3

Kitchen Essentials for Type A Dieters

For Type A dieters, having the appropriate kitchen necessities on hand is crucial to preparing wholesome meals that suit their blood type. The following is a list of kitchen necessities designed with Type A dieters in mind:

- Investing in sturdy cutting boards composed of plastic or bamboo can help you slice fruits, vegetables, and proteins with ease. To avoid cross-contamination, think about keeping raw meats and veggies on different cutting boards.

- High-quality knives are necessary for accurate and effective food preparation. A set should include a chef's knife, paring knife, and serrated knife. Chopping and slicing becomes safer and simpler with sharp knives.

- Food processors and blenders are multipurpose kitchen appliances that may be used to chop vegetables, mix sauces, prepare smoothies, and puree soups. Select a model for optimal functionality that comes with several attachments.

Vegetable Spiralizer: A useful kitchen tool, a vegetable spiralizer transforms veggies like sweet potatoes, carrots, and zucchini into strands that resemble noodles, ideal for making colorful and healthful salads, stir-fries, and pasta substitutes.

Steamer Basket: Steam cooking retains the nutrients and tastes of veggies since it's a gentle cooking technique. Vegetables steam quickly and effortlessly with the help of a steamer basket, producing soft, colorful greens.

Cookware that doesn't stick: For Type A dieters who want lighter cooking techniques, non-stick pots and pans are perfect since they use less oil while cooking. When cooking, choose non-toxic, PFOA-free products for greater safety and wellness.

Salad Spinner: For efficient and speedy washing and drying of leafy greens, herbs, and vegetables, a salad spinner is needed. It takes out extra water so that salads are always crisp and fresh.

Purchase a collection of glass mason jars or containers to store homemade sauces, dressings, snacks, and meals that are prepared in bulk. Glass containers are strong, safe for the environment, and devoid of the dangerous chemicals included in plastic.

Measuring Cups and Spoons: Precise ingredient portioning and recipe adherence depend heavily on accurate measuring cups and spoons. For maximum adaptability, look for a set that contains both liquid and dry measurements.

Herb Keeper: By maintaining the ideal humidity and ventilation, an herb keeper, also known as an herb storage container, helps preserve the freshness of delicate herbs like basil, cilantro, and parsley. This keeps herbs bright and delicious for longer.

Vegetable Storage Bags or Containers: Store fruits and vegetables in breathable produce bags or containers that are designed to control humidity and keep food from spoiling to increase its shelf life. As a result, less food is wasted and products remain fresher for longer.

Cookbook Stand or Holder: Using a cookbook stand or holder will make it simple to reach your preferred blood type diet cookbook or recipe cards while cooking. You may follow recipes hands-free by using it to keep pages open and erect.

Having these basic kitchen tools on hand can make meal prep easier and enable Type A dieters to make delicious, nutritious meals that promote their well-being. Depending on your blood type, cooking may be a fulfilling and pleasurable activity if you have the correct supplies and instruments.

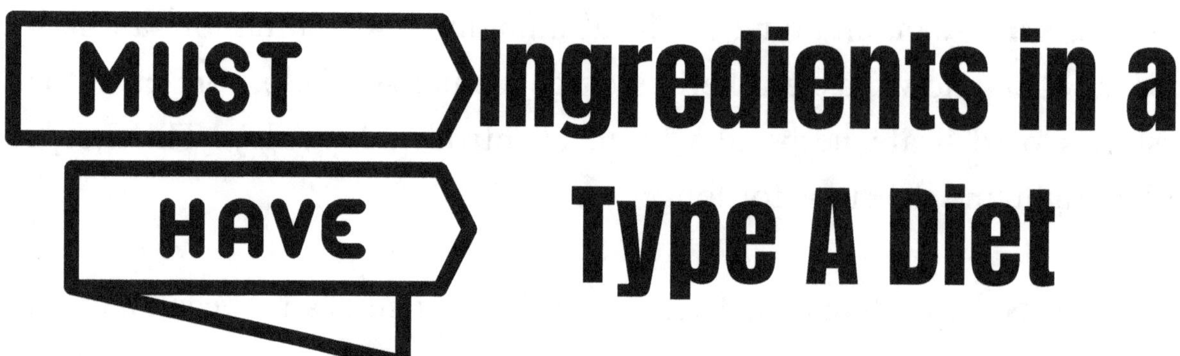

It's important for Type A personalities to include the correct nutrients in their diet if they want to maximize their health and well-being. The following is a list of essential elements for a Type A diet:

Leafy Greens: High in vitamins, minerals, and antioxidants are leafy greens including spinach, kale, Swiss chard, and collard greens. They promote general health and energy while offering crucial minerals including iron, vitamin K, and folate.

Colorful Vegetables: Include bell peppers, carrots, beets, sweet potatoes, and squash in your diet, among other colorful veggies. Packed with vitamins, minerals, and phytonutrients that lower inflammation and strengthen the immune system are these veggies.

Plant-Based Proteins: Choose legumes, chickpeas, tofu, tempeh, and beans as your plant-based protein sources. These high-protein meals provide the essential amino acids required for muscle development and repair and are consistent with a Type A diet.

Whole Grains: As the base of your meals, use whole grains such as millet, quinoa, brown rice, barley, and oats. The substantial fiber content of whole grains helps to normalize blood sugar levels and promotes digestive health.

Good Fats: Include foods like avocados, olive oil, nuts, and seeds in your diet as sources of good fats. These fats provide vital fatty acids that enhance heart health, lower inflammation, and boost brain function.

Fresh Fruits: Savor a range of fresh fruits, such as melons, apples, berries, grapes, and citrus fruits. Fruits help curb cravings for sweets due to their inherent sweetness and abundance of vitamins, minerals, and antioxidants.

Herbs and Spices: Use herbs and spices like turmeric, cinnamon, cumin, garlic, ginger, parsley, cilantro, and basil to enhance the taste of your food. Spices and herbs provide food with more nuance and richness without the use of harmful or excessively salty ingredients.

Fermented Foods: To improve digestion and gut health, include fermented foods in your diet, such as kimchi, yogurt, kefir, and sauerkraut. Good probiotics found in fermented foods support a balanced population of gut flora.

Sea Vegetables: To increase mineral intake and improve thyroid function, include sea vegetables like nori, kombu, dulse, and wakame in your diet. Iodine, iron, calcium, and other trace elements that are vital to health are abundant in sea veggies.

Green Tea: Drink green tea to hydrate and nourish your body. It contains antioxidants that help maintain healthy cells and the immune system. Additionally linked to several health advantages, such as enhanced heart health and metabolism, is green tea.

These essential components will help you prepare nutritious meals that meet your specific nutritional demands and advance your general health and well-being while adhering to a Type A diet. Try a variety of combos and recipes to keep your meals enjoyable and engaging while enjoying the advantages of a blood-type-specific diet.

CHAPTER

4

BREAKFAST RECIPES

Quinoa Breakfast Bowl

Calories	Protein	Carbohydrates	Fiber	Fat
300	8g	50g	7g	5g

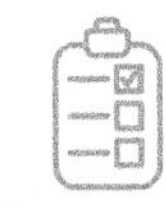 5 minutes

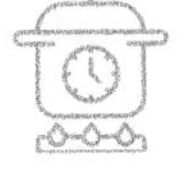 15 minutes

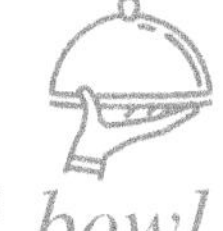 1 bowl

INGREDIENTS

Cooked quinoa
almond milk
fresh berries
sliced banana
chia seeds
honey.

INSTRUCTIONS

Combine cooked quinoa with almond milk, top with fresh berries, sliced banana, chia seeds, and drizzle with honey.

Spinach and Feta Omelette

Calories	Protein	Carbohydrates	Fiber	Fat
250	18g	5g	3g	18g

 5 minutes

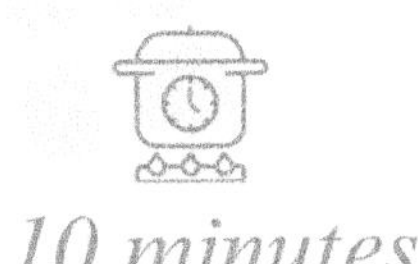 10 minutes

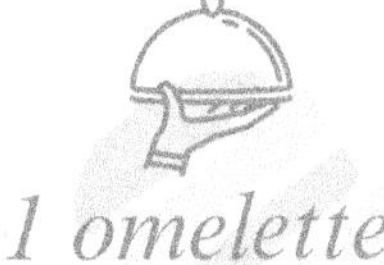 1 omelette

INGREDIENTS

Eggs,
spinach, feta
cheese,
cherry
tomatoes,
olive oil.

INSTRUCTIONS

Whisk eggs, sauté spinach in olive oil, add whisked eggs, top with feta cheese and cherry tomatoes, fold omelette, and cook until set.

Greek Yogurt Parfait

Calories	Protein	Carbohydrates	Fiber	Fat
300	15g	40g	5g	10g

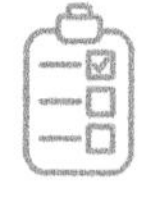 5 minutes

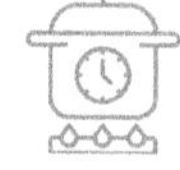 5 minutes

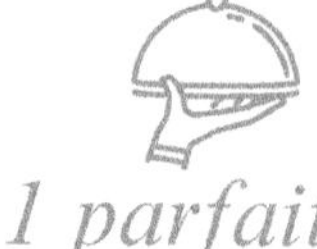 1 parfait

INGREDIENTS

Greek yogurt, granola, fresh berries, honey

INSTRUCTIONS

Layer Greek yogurt, granola, and fresh berries in a glass, drizzle with honey

Almond Butter Banana Toast

Calories	Protein	Carbohydrates	Fiber	Fat
200	6g	30g	5g	8g

 5 minutes

 5 minutes

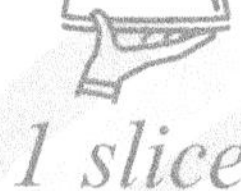 1 slice

INGREDIENTS

Whole grain bread, almond butter, sliced banana, cinnamon.

INSTRUCTIONS

Toast whole grain bread, spread almond butter, top with sliced banana, and sprinkle with cinnamon.

Berry Smoothie Bowl

Calories	Protein	Carbohydrates	Fiber	Fat
250	5g	40g	10g	5g

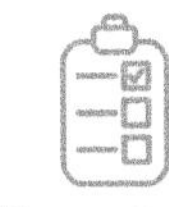

5 minutes

5 minutes

1 bowl

INGREDIENTS

Frozen mixed berries, almond milk, spinach, banana, chia seeds.

INSTRUCTIONS

Blend frozen berries, almond milk, spinach, and banana until smooth, pour into a bowl, and top with chia seeds.

Avocado Toast with Poached Egg

Calories	Protein	Carbohydrates	Fiber	Fat
250	10g	20g	5g	15g

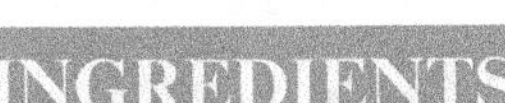

5 minutes

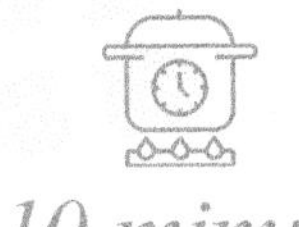

10 minutes

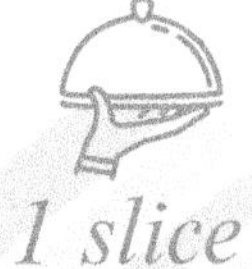

1 slice

INGREDIENTS

Whole grain bread, avocado, eggs, cherry tomatoes, olive oil.

INSTRUCTIONS

Toast whole grain bread, mash avocado, poach egg, top toast with mashed avocado, poached egg, and cherry tomatoes, drizzle with olive oil.

Chia Seed Pudding

Calories	Protein	Carbohydrates	Fiber	Fat
200	5g	20g	10g	10g

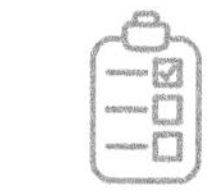

5 minutes (plus overnight refrigeration)

5 minutes

1 pudding cup

INGREDIENTS

Chia seeds, almond milk, vanilla extract, maple syrup, fresh fruit.

INSTRUCTIONS

Mix chia seeds, almond milk, vanilla extract, and maple syrup, refrigerate overnight, top with fresh fruit before serving.

Vegetable Frittata

Calories	Protein	Carbohydrates	Fiber	Fat
150	10g	5g	2g	10g

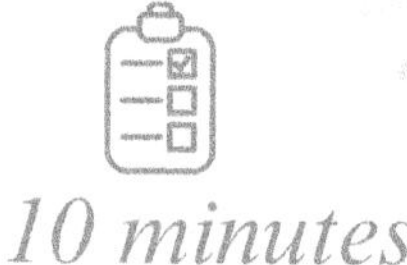

10 minutes

20 minutes

1 slice

INGREDIENTS

Eggs, spinach, bell peppers, onion, cherry tomatoes, feta cheese, olive oil.

INSTRUCTIONS

Sauté vegetables in olive oil, whisk eggs, pour over vegetables, top with feta cheese, bake until set.

Coconut Yogurt with Mango Slices

Calories	Protein	Carbohydrates	Fiber	Fat
200	5g	30g	5g	8g

5 minutes

5 minutes

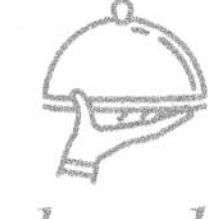

1 bowl

INGREDIENTS

Coconut yogurt, fresh mango, shredded coconut, honey

INSTRUCTIONS

Top coconut yogurt with fresh mango slices, shredded coconut, and drizzle with honey.

Millet Porridge with Berries

Calories	Protein	Carbohydrates	Fiber	Fat
300	g	50g	8g	5g

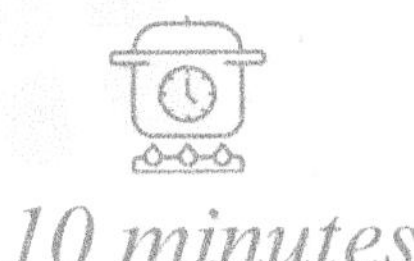

5 minutes

10 minutes

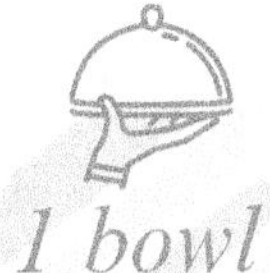

1 bowl

INGREDIENTS

Cooked millet, almond milk, cinnamon, fresh berries, honey.

INSTRUCTIONS

Heat cooked millet with almond milk and cinnamon, top with fresh berries, and drizzle with honey

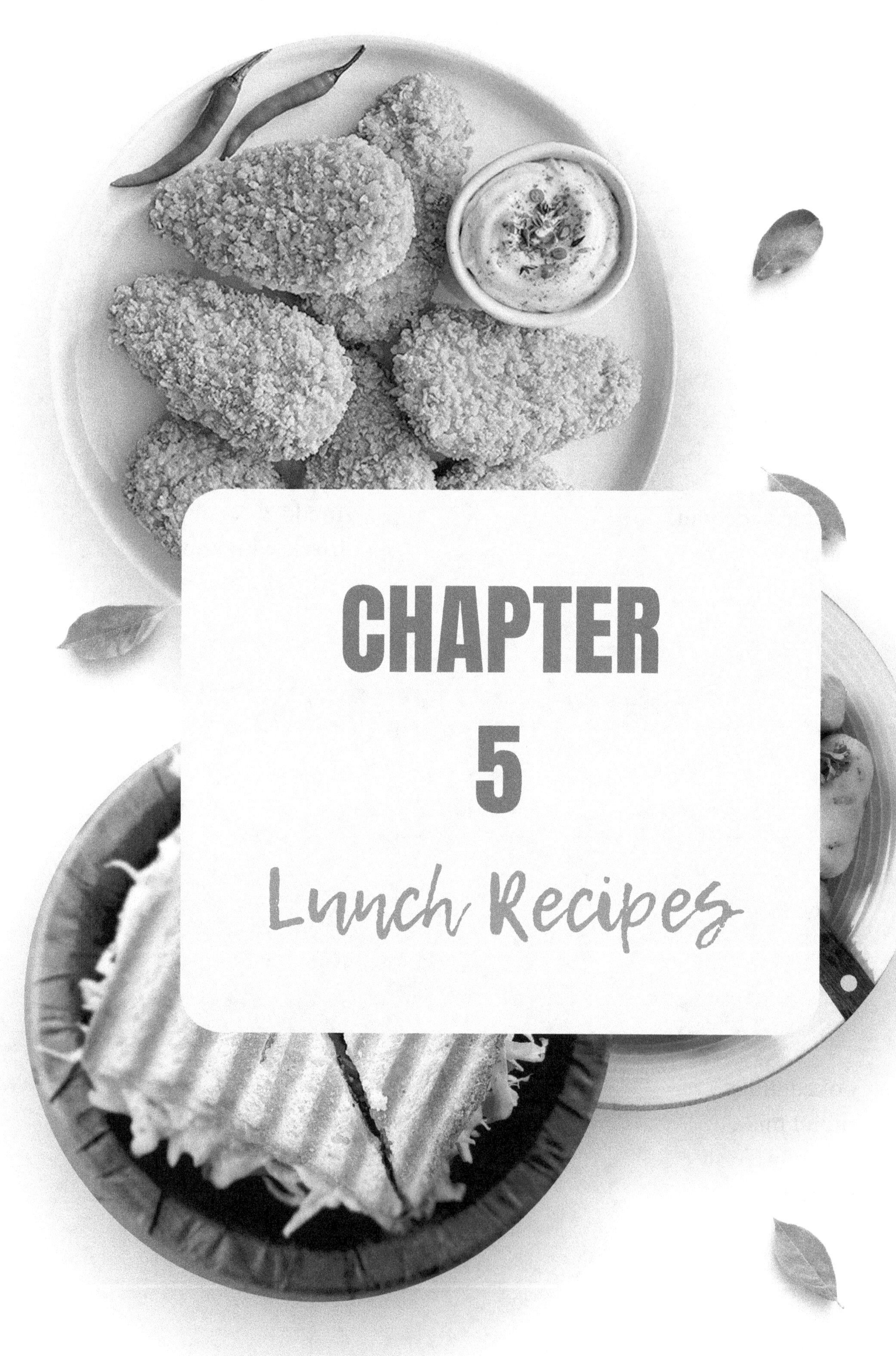

CHAPTER
5
Lunch Recipes

Quinoa Salad with Chickpeas and Vegetables

Calories	Protein	Carbohydrates	Fiber	Fat
250	9g	38g	7g	8g

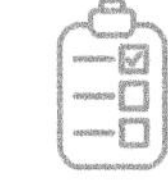 10 minutes

 20 minutes

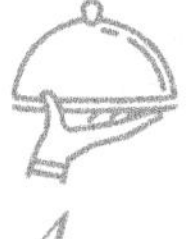 4

INGREDIENTS

1. 1 cup cooked quinoa
2. 1 cup canned chickpeas, rinsed and drained
3. 1 cup diced cucumber
4. 1 cup cherry tomatoes, halved
5. 1/2 cup chopped bell pepper
6. 1/4 cup chopped fresh parsley
7. 2 tablespoons lemon juice
8. 1 tablespoon olive oil
9. Salt and pepper to taste

INSTRUCTIONS

1. In a large bowl, combine cooked quinoa, chickpeas, cucumber, tomatoes, bell pepper, and parsley.
2. In a small bowl, whisk together lemon juice, olive oil, salt, and pepper. Pour over the quinoa mixture and toss to combine.
3. Serve chilled or at room temperature

Lentil and Vegetable Soup

Calories	Protein	Carbohydrates	Fiber	Fat
220	13g	38g	10g	10g

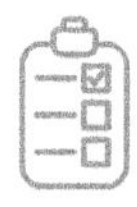 10 minutes

 30 minutes

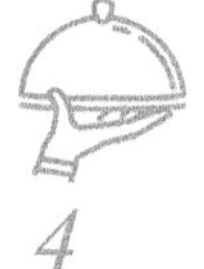 4

INGREDIENTS

1. 1 cup dry green lentils
2. 4 cups vegetable broth
3. 1 onion, diced
4. 2 carrots, diced
5. 2 celery stalks, diced
6. 2 cloves garlic, minced
7. 1 teaspoon dried thyme
8. Salt and pepper to taste

INSTRUCTIONS

1. In a large pot, combine lentils, vegetable broth, onion, carrots, celery, garlic, and thyme.
2. Bring to a boil, then reduce heat and simmer for 20-25 minutes until lentils are tender.
3. Season with salt and pepper to taste before serving.

Tofu Stir-Fry with Broccoli and Bell Peppers

Calories	Protein	Carbohydrates	Fiber	Fat
280	18g	22g	14g	6g

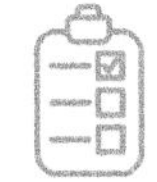

15 minutes

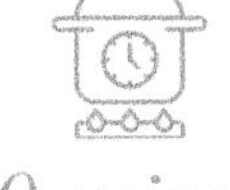

20 minutes

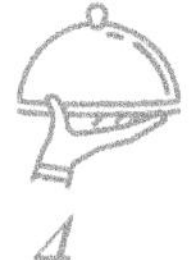

4

INGREDIENTS

1. 1 block firm tofu, pressed and cubed
2. 2 cups broccoli florets
3. 1 red bell pepper, sliced
4. 1 yellow bell pepper, sliced
5. 2 tablespoons soy sauce
6. 1 tablespoon sesame oil
7. 2 cloves garlic, minced
8. 1 teaspoon grated ginger
9. Cooked brown rice or quinoa for serving

INSTRUCTIONS

1. Heat sesame oil in a large skillet over medium heat. Add tofu cubes and cook until golden brown on all sides. Remove from skillet and set aside.
2. In the same skillet, add broccoli florets, bell peppers, garlic, and ginger. Stir-fry for 5-7 minutes until vegetables are tender-crisp.
3. Return tofu to the skillet, add soy sauce, and toss to combine. Cook for an additional 2-3 minutes.
4. Serve tofu stir-fry over cooked brown rice or quinoa.

Chickpea and Avocado Wrap

Calories	Protein	Carbohydrates	Fiber	Fat
320	12g	45g	12g	10g

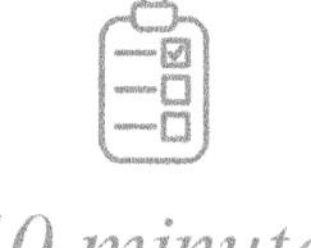 10 minutes

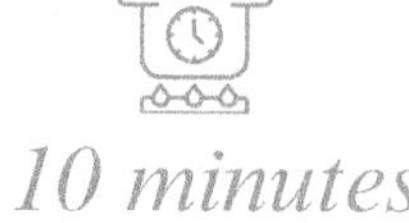 10 minutes

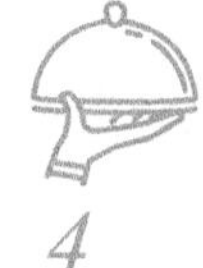 4

INGREDIENTS

1. 1 (15 oz) can chickpeas, drained and rinsed
2. 1 ripe avocado, mashed
3. 1/4 cup diced red onion
4. 1/4 cup chopped fresh cilantro
5. Juice of 1 lime
6. Salt and pepper to taste
7. 4 whole grain wraps or tortillas
8. Spinach or lettuce leaves for filling

INSTRUCTIONS

1. In a bowl, combine mashed avocado, chickpeas, red onion, cilantro, lime juice, salt, and pepper. Mash lightly with a fork until well mixed.
2. Lay out wraps or tortillas and divide chickpea-avocado mixture evenly among them. Top with spinach or lettuce leaves.
3. Roll up wraps tightly, slice in half, and serve immediately

Mediterranean Quinoa Bowl

Calories	Protein	Carbohydrates	Fiber	Fat
280	8g	30g	14g	6g

10 minutes *15 minutes* 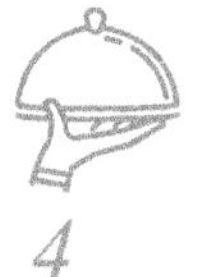 4

1. 1 cup cooked quinoa
2. 1 cup diced cucumber
3. 1 cup cherry tomatoes, halved
4. 1/2 cup sliced Kalamata olives
5. 1/4 cup crumbled feta cheese
6. 2 tablespoons chopped fresh parsley
7. 1 tablespoon extra virgin olive oil
8. Juice of 1 lemon
9. Salt and pepper to taste

1. In a bowl, combine cooked quinoa, cucumber, cherry tomatoes, olives, feta cheese, and parsley.
2. Drizzle with olive oil and lemon juice, then season with salt and pepper to taste. Toss to combine.
3. Serve quinoa mixture in bowls and enjoy immediately.

Spinach and Strawberry Salad with Balsamic Vinaigrette

Calories	Protein	Carbohydrates	Fiber	Fat
150	4g	12g	10g	4g

 10 minutes

 10 minutes

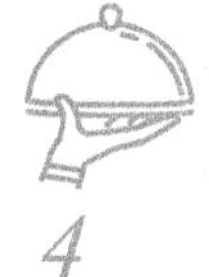 4

INGREDIENTS

1. 6 cups baby spinach
2. 1 cup sliced strawberries
3. 1/4 cup sliced almonds
4. 1/4 cup crumbled goat cheese
5. 2 tablespoons balsamic vinegar
6. 1 tablespoon extra virgin olive oil
7. 1 teaspoon honey
8. Salt and pepper to taste

INSTRUCTIONS

1. In a large bowl, combine baby spinach, sliced strawberries, sliced almonds, and crumbled goat cheese.
2. In a small bowl, whisk together balsamic vinegar, olive oil, honey, salt, and pepper to make the vinaigrette.
3. Drizzle the vinaigrette over the salad and toss gently to coat.
4. Serve immediately as a refreshing lunch option.

Veggie and Hummus Wrap

Calories	Protein	Carbohydrates	Fiber	Fat
220	8g	32g	7g	7g

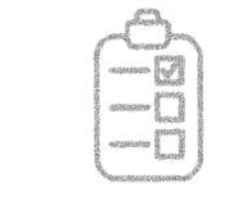 10 minutes

 10 minutes

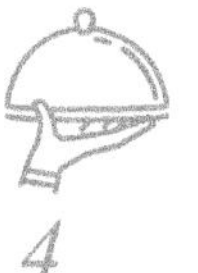 4

INGREDIENTS

1. 4 whole grain wraps or tortillas
2. 1/2 cup hummus
3. 1 cup shredded carrots
4. 1 cup thinly sliced cucumber
5. 1 cup baby spinach leaves
6. 1/4 cup sliced red onion
7. Salt and pepper to taste

INSTRUCTIONS

1. Lay out wraps or tortillas and spread a layer of hummus evenly over each one.
2. Divide shredded carrots, sliced cucumber, baby spinach, and red onion among the wraps.
3. Season with salt and pepper to taste.
4. Roll up wraps tightly, slice in half, and serve immediately.

Greek Lentil Salad

Calories	Protein	Carbohydrates	Fiber	Fat
220	13g	35g	10g	12g

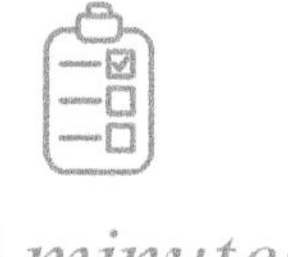 10 minutes

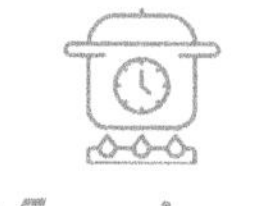 25 minutes

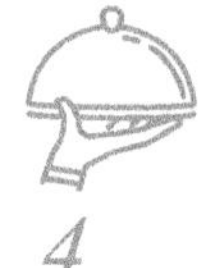 4

1. 1 cup dry green lentils
2. 2 cups water or vegetable broth
3. 1 cucumber, diced
4. 1 cup cherry tomatoes, halved
5. 1/4 cup diced red onion
6. 1/4 cup chopped fresh parsley
7. 1/4 cup crumbled feta cheese
8. 2 tablespoons extra virgin olive oil
9. 2 tablespoons red wine vinegar
10. Salt and pepper to taste

1. Rinse lentils under cold water and drain. Place lentils in a pot with water or vegetable broth and bring to a boil.
2. Reduce heat, cover, and simmer for 20-25 minutes until lentils are tender. Drain any excess liquid and let cool.
3. In a large bowl, combine cooked lentils, cucumber, cherry tomatoes, red onion, parsley, and feta cheese.
4. Drizzle olive oil and red wine vinegar over the salad, then season with salt and pepper to taste. Toss to combine.
5. Serve chilled or at room temperature.

Veggie and Tofu Stir-Fry with Brown Rice

Calories	Protein	Carbohydrates	Fiber	Fat
320	15g	40g	12g	8g

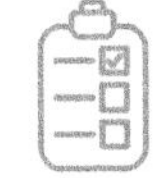 15 minutes

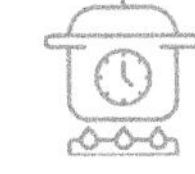 20 minutes

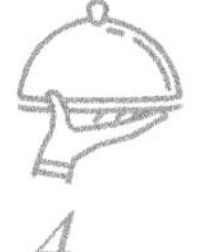 4

INGREDIENTS

1. 1 block firm tofu, pressed and cubed
2. 2 cups mixed vegetables (broccoli, bell peppers, carrots, snap peas)
3. 2 tablespoons soy saucc
4. 1 tablespoon hoisin sauce
5. 1 tablespoon sesame oil
6. 2 cloves garlic, minced
7. 1 teaspoon grated ginger
8. Cooked brown rice for serving

INSTRUCTIONS

1. Heat sesame oil in a large skillet over medium heat. Add tofu cubes and cook until golden brown on all sides. Remove from skillet and set aside.
2. In the same skillet, add mixed vegetables, garlic, and ginger. Stir-fry for 5-7 minutes until vegetables are tender-crisp.
3. Return tofu to the skillet, add soy sauce and hoisin sauce, and toss to combine. Cook for an additional 2-3 minutes.
4. Serve tofu stir-fry over cooked brown rice.

Mediterranean Chickpea Salad

Calories	Protein	Carbohydrates	Fiber	Fat
240	10g	30g	10g	8g

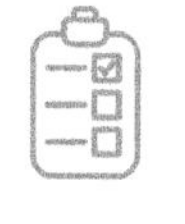

10 minutes

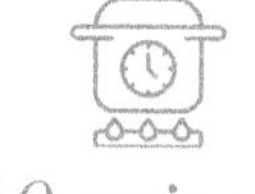

10 minutes

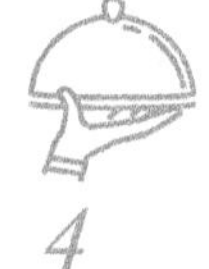

4

INGREDIENTS

1. 1 (15 oz) can chickpeas, drained and rinsed
2. 1 cucumber, diced
3. 1 cup cherry tomatoes, halved
4. 1/4 cup diced red onion
5. 1/4 cup chopped fresh parsley
6. 2 tablespoons extra virgin olive oil
7. 2 tablespoons red wine vinegar
8. Juice of 1 lemon
9. Salt and pepper to taste

INSTRUCTIONS

1. In a large bowl, combine chickpeas, cucumber, cherry tomatoes, red onion, and parsley.
2. In a small bowl, whisk together olive oil, red wine vinegar, lemon juice, salt, and pepper to make the dressing.
3. Pour the dressing over the salad and toss gently to coat.
4. Serve chilled or at room temperature.

CHAPTER 6

HEALTHY DINNER IDEAS

Quinoa-Stuffed Bell Peppers

Calories	Protein	Carbohydrates	Fiber	Fat
320	13g	56g	5g	12g

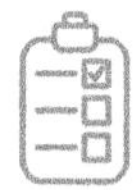 15 minutes

 30-35 minutes

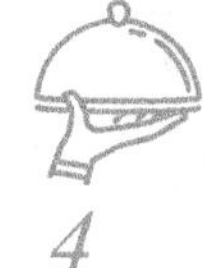 4

INGREDIENTS

1. 4 bell peppers (any color)
2. 1 cup quinoa, cooked
3. 1 can black beans, drained and rinsed
4. 1 cup corn kernels
5. 1 cup diced tomatoes
6. 1/2 cup chopped onion
7. 2 cloves garlic, minced
8. 1 teaspoon cumin
9. 1/2 teaspoon chili powder
10. Salt and pepper to taste
11. 1/2 cup shredded cheese (optional)

INSTRUCTIONS

1. Preheat the oven to 375°F (190°C). Cut the tops off the bell peppers and remove the seeds and membranes.
2. In a large bowl, combine cooked quinoa, black beans, corn, diced tomatoes, onion, garlic, cumin, chili powder, salt, and pepper.
3. Stuff each bell pepper with the quinoa mixture and place them in a baking dish. If using cheese, sprinkle it on top of each stuffed pepper.
4. Cover the baking dish with foil and bake for 25-30 minutes, or until the peppers are tender.
5. Remove the foil and bake for an additional 5 minutes to melt the cheese (if using).
6. Serve hot and enjoy!

Lemon Herb Baked Salmon

Calories	Protein	Carbohydrates	Fiber	Fat
280	30g	2g	16g	1g

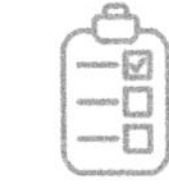

10 minutes

12-15 minutes

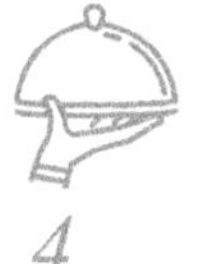

4

INGREDIENTS

1. 4 salmon fillets
2. 2 tablespoons olive oil
3. 2 tablespoons lemon juice
4. 2 cloves garlic, minced
5. 1 teaspoon dried thyme
6. 1 teaspoon dried rosemary
7. Salt and pepper to taste
8. Lemon slices for garnish

INSTRUCTIONS

1. Preheat the oven to 375°F (190°C). Place salmon fillets on a baking sheet lined with parchment paper.
2. In a small bowl, whisk together olive oil, lemon juice, minced garlic, dried thyme, dried rosemary, salt, and pepper.
3. Pour the mixture over the salmon fillets, making sure they are evenly coated.
4. Bake in the preheated oven for 12-15 minutes, or until the salmon is cooked through and flakes easily with a fork.
5. Garnish with lemon slices and serve hot.

Mediterranean Chickpea Salad

Calories	Protein	Carbohydrates	Fiber	Fat
240	8g	27g	12g	7g

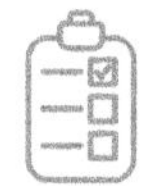 15 minutes

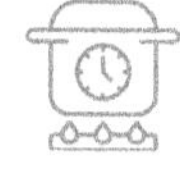 10 minutes (if using canned chickpeas)

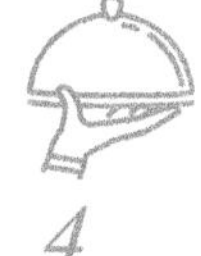 4

INGREDIENTS

1. 2 cups cooked chickpeas (or 1 can, drained and rinsed)
2. 1 cup cherry tomatoes, halved
3. 1 cucumber, diced
4. 1/2 red onion, thinly sliced
5. 1/4 cup chopped fresh parsley
6. 1/4 cup chopped fresh mint
7. 2 tablespoons olive oil
8. 2 tablespoons lemon juice
9. 1 teaspoon dried oregano
10. Salt and pepper to taste
11. Crumbled feta cheese for garnish (optional)

INSTRUCTIONS

1. In a large bowl, combine cooked chickpeas, cherry tomatoes, cucumber, red onion, parsley, and mint.
2. In a small bowl, whisk together olive oil, lemon juice, dried oregano, salt, and pepper.
3. Pour the dressing over the chickpea mixture and toss until well coated.
4. Garnish with crumbled feta cheese (if using) and serve chilled or at room temperature.

Vegetable Stir-Fry with Tofu

Calories	Protein	Carbohydrates	Fiber	Fat
220	16g	14g	12g	5g

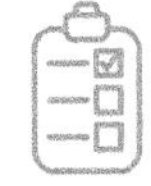 15 minutes

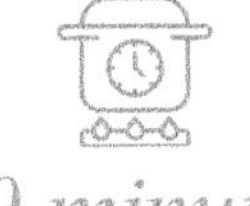 20 minutes

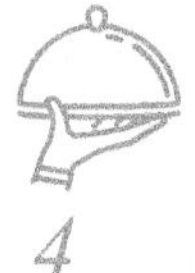 4

INGREDIENTS

1. 14 oz (400g) extra-firm tofu, pressed and cubed
2. 2 cups broccoli florets
3. 1 red bell pepper, sliced
4. 1 yellow bell pepper, sliced
5. 1 cup snap peas
6. 1 carrot, julienned
7. 2 cloves garlic, minced
8. 2 tablespoons soy sauce
9. 1 tablespoon sesame oil
10. 1 tablespoon rice vinegar
11. 1 teaspoon ginger, grated
12. 2 green onions, chopped (for garnish)

Cooked brown rice or quinoa for serving

INSTRUCTIONS

1. In a large skillet or wok, heat sesame oil over medium-high heat. Add cubed tofu and cook until golden brown on all sides. Remove tofu from skillet and set aside.
2. In the same skillet, add a bit more sesame oil if needed. Add garlic and ginger, and cook for 1 minute.
3. Add broccoli, bell peppers, snap peas, and carrot to the skillet. Stir-fry for 5-7 minutes, or until vegetables are tender-crisp.
4. Return tofu to the skillet. Add soy sauce and rice vinegar, and toss until everything is well coated.
5. Serve stir-fry over cooked brown rice or quinoa. Garnish with chopped green onions and enjoy!

Lentil and Vegetable Curry

Calories	Protein	Carbohydrates	Fiber	Fat
360	14g	35g	19g	11g

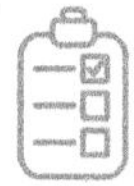 15 minutes

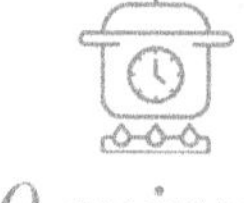 30 minutes

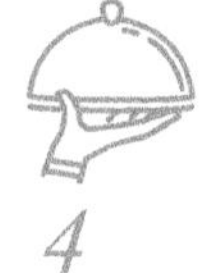 4

INGREDIENTS

1. 1 cup dried green lentils, rinsed and drained
2. 1 onion, diced
3. 2 cloves garlic, minced
4. 1 tablespoon grated ginger
5. 2 carrots, diced
6. 1 bell pepper, diced
7. 1 zucchini, diced
8. 1 can (14 oz) diced tomatoes
9. 1 can (14 oz) coconut milk
10. 2 tablespoons curry powder
11. 1 teaspoon turmeric
12. Salt and pepper to taste
13. Fresh cilantro for garnish
14. Cooked brown rice for serving

INSTRUCTIONS

1. In a large pot, heat olive oil over medium heat. Add diced onion, garlic, and grated ginger. Cook until softened and fragrant, about 5 minutes.
2. Add diced carrots, bell pepper, and zucchini to the pot. Cook for another 5 minutes, or until vegetables start to soften.
3. Stir in curry powder and turmeric, and cook for 1 minute until fragrant.
4. Add rinsed lentils, diced tomatoes, and coconut milk to the pot. Bring to a simmer and let cook for 20-25 minutes, or until lentils are tender.
5. Season with salt and pepper to taste. Serve curry over cooked brown rice and garnish with fresh cilantro.

Grilled Vegetable Skewers

Calories	Protein	Carbohydrates	Fiber	Fat
140	4g	14g	8g	4g

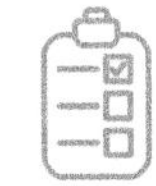 15 minutes

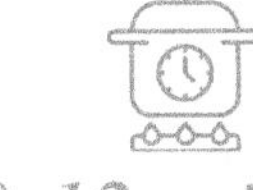 10-12 minutes

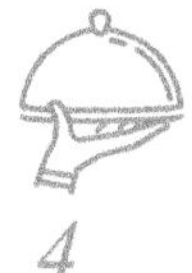 4

INGREDIENTS

1. 2 zucchinis, sliced into rounds
2. 1 yellow squash, sliced into rounds
3. 1 red onion, cut into chunks
4. 1 bell pepper, cut into chunks
5. 1 cup cherry tomatoes
6. 8 oz (225g) mushrooms, whole or halved
7. 2 tablespoons olive oil
8. 2 cloves garlic, minced
9. 1 teaspoon dried oregano
10. 1 teaspoon dried thyme
11. Salt and pepper to taste
12. Wooden skewers, soaked in water

INSTRUCTIONS

1. Preheat the grill to medium-high heat.
2. In a large bowl, toss zucchini, yellow squash, red onion, bell pepper, cherry tomatoes, and mushrooms with olive oil, minced garlic, dried oregano, dried thyme, salt, and pepper.
3. Thread the marinated vegetables onto the soaked wooden skewers, alternating between different vegetables.
4. Place the skewers on the preheated grill and cook for 10-12 minutes, turning occasionally, or until vegetables are tender and lightly charred.
5. Remove skewers from the grill and serve hot as a delicious and colorful side dish.

Eggplant and Chickpea Tagine

Calories	Protein	Carbohydrates	Fiber	Fat
180	6g	28g	5g	9g

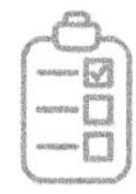 15 minutes

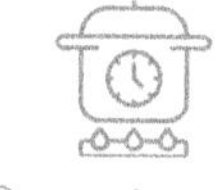 30 minutes

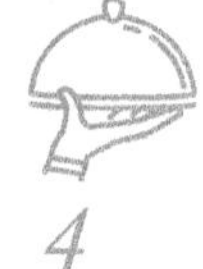 4

INGREDIENTS

1. 1 eggplant, cubed
2. 1 can (14 oz) chickpeas, drained and rinsed
3. 1 onion, diced
4. 2 cloves garlic, minced
5. 1 can (14 oz) diced tomatoes
6. 1 cup vegetable broth
7. 1 teaspoon ground cumin
8. 1 teaspoon ground coriander
9. 1/2 teaspoon ground cinnamon
10. Salt and pepper to taste
11. Fresh cilantro for garnish
12. Cooked couscous for serving

INSTRUCTIONS

1. Heat olive oil in a large pot or tagine over medium heat. Add diced onion and minced garlic, and cook until softened and fragrant, about 5 minutes.
2. Add cubed eggplant to the pot and cook for another 5 minutes, stirring occasionally.
3. Stir in ground cumin, ground coriander, and ground cinnamon, and cook for 1 minute until fragrant.
4. Add diced tomatoes, drained chickpeas, and vegetable broth to the pot. Season with salt and pepper to taste.
5. Bring the mixture to a simmer, then reduce heat to low and let simmer, covered, for 20-25 minutes, or until eggplant is tender and flavors have melded.
6. Serve tagine over cooked couscous and garnish with fresh cilantro.

Spinach and Mushroom Quiche

Calories	Protein	Carbohydrates	Fiber	Fat
280	12g	18g	18g	2g

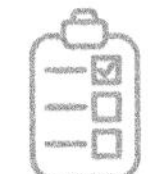

20 minutes

35-40 minutes

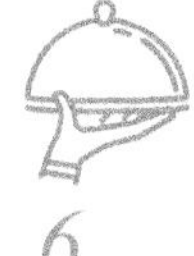

6

INGREDIENTS

1. 1 store-bought or homemade pie crust
2. 6 large eggs
3. 1 cup milk (dairy or plant-based)
4. 2 cups fresh spinach, chopped
5. 1 cup mushrooms, sliced
6. 1/2 cup shredded cheese (such as Swiss or feta)
7. 1/4 cup diced onion
8. 2 cloves garlic, minced
9. 1 tablespoon olive oil
10. Salt and pepper to taste

INSTRUCTIONS

- Preheat the oven to 375°F (190°C). Roll out the pie crust and press it into a pie dish, trimming any excess crust around the edges.
- In a skillet, heat olive oil over medium heat. Add diced onion and minced garlic, and cook until softened and fragrant, about 5 minutes.
- Add sliced mushrooms to the skillet and cook until they release their moisture and start to brown, about 5-7 minutes.
- Add chopped spinach to the skillet and cook until wilted, about 2-3 minutes. Remove from heat and let cool slightly.
- In a large bowl, whisk together eggs and milk until well combined. Season with salt and pepper to taste.
- Spread the cooked mushroom and spinach mixture evenly over the bottom of the prepared pie crust. Sprinkle shredded cheese on top.
- Pour the egg mixture over the vegetables and cheese in the pie crust.
- Bake in the preheated oven for 35-40 minutes, or until the center is set and the top is golden brown.
- Remove from the oven and let cool for a few minutes before slicing and serving.

Turkey and Vegetable Lettuce Wraps

Calories	Protein	Carbohydrates	Fiber	Fat
240	25g	10g	11g	2g

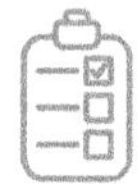

10 minutes

15 minutes

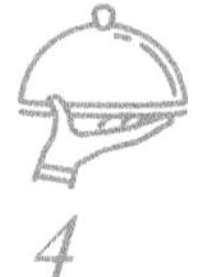

4

INGREDIENTS

1. 1 lb (450g) lean ground turkey
2. 1 tablespoon olive oil
3. 2 cloves garlic, minced
4. 1 teaspoon grated ginger
5. 1 bell pepper, diced
6. 1 carrot, grated
7. 1/2 cup sliced water chestnuts
8. 1/4 cup hoisin sauce
9. 2 tablespoons soy sauce
10. 1 tablespoon rice vinegar
11. 1 teaspoon sesame oil
12. Salt and pepper to taste
13. Butter lettuce leaves for wrapping

INSTRUCTIONS

1. In a large skillet, heat olive oil over medium heat. Add minced garlic and grated ginger, and cook for 1 minute until fragrant.
2. Add ground turkey to the skillet and cook until browned and cooked through, breaking it up with a spoon as it cooks.
3. Add diced bell pepper, grated carrot, and sliced water chestnuts to the skillet. Cook for another 3-4 minutes, or until vegetables are tender-crisp.
4. In a small bowl, whisk together hoisin sauce, soy sauce, rice vinegar, and sesame oil. Pour the sauce over the turkey and vegetable mixture in the skillet.
5. Stir to coat everything evenly with the sauce. Season with salt and pepper to taste.
6. Remove from heat and spoon the turkey and vegetable mixture onto butter lettuce leaves. Roll up the leaves to form wraps and serve immediately.

Vegetable and Tofu Stir-Fry with Brown Rice

Calories	Protein	Carbohydrates	Fiber	Fat
280	15g	16g	5g	18g

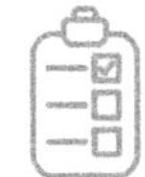

15 minutes

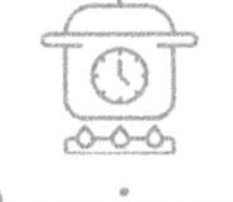

20 minutes

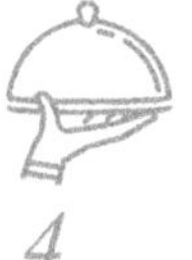

4

INGREDIENTS

1. 14 oz (400g) extra-firm tofu, pressed and cubed
2. 2 tablespoons soy sauce
3. 1 tablespoon sesame oil
4. 1 tablespoon cornstarch
5. 2 tablespoons olive oil
6. 2 cloves garlic, minced
7. 1 teaspoon grated ginger
8. 2 cups broccoli florets
9. 1 red bell pepper, sliced
10. 1 yellow bell pepper, sliced
11. 1 cup snap peas
12. 1 carrot, julienned
13. Cooked brown rice for serving

INSTRUCTIONS

1. In a bowl, combine cubed tofu with soy sauce, sesame oil, and cornstarch. Toss to coat the tofu evenly, then let marinate for 10-15 minutes.
2. Heat olive oil in a large skillet or wok over medium-high heat. Add minced garlic and grated ginger, and cook for 1 minute until fragrant.
3. Add marinated tofu to the skillet and cook until golden brown on all sides. Remove tofu from skillet and set aside.
4. In the same skillet, add a bit more olive oil if needed. Add broccoli, bell peppers, snap peas, and julienned carrot. Stir-fry for 5-7 minutes, or until vegetables are tender-crisp.
5. Return tofu to the skillet and toss with the vegetables until heated through.
6. Serve stir-fry over cooked brown rice and enjoy!

CHAPTER
7
SNACK RECIPES

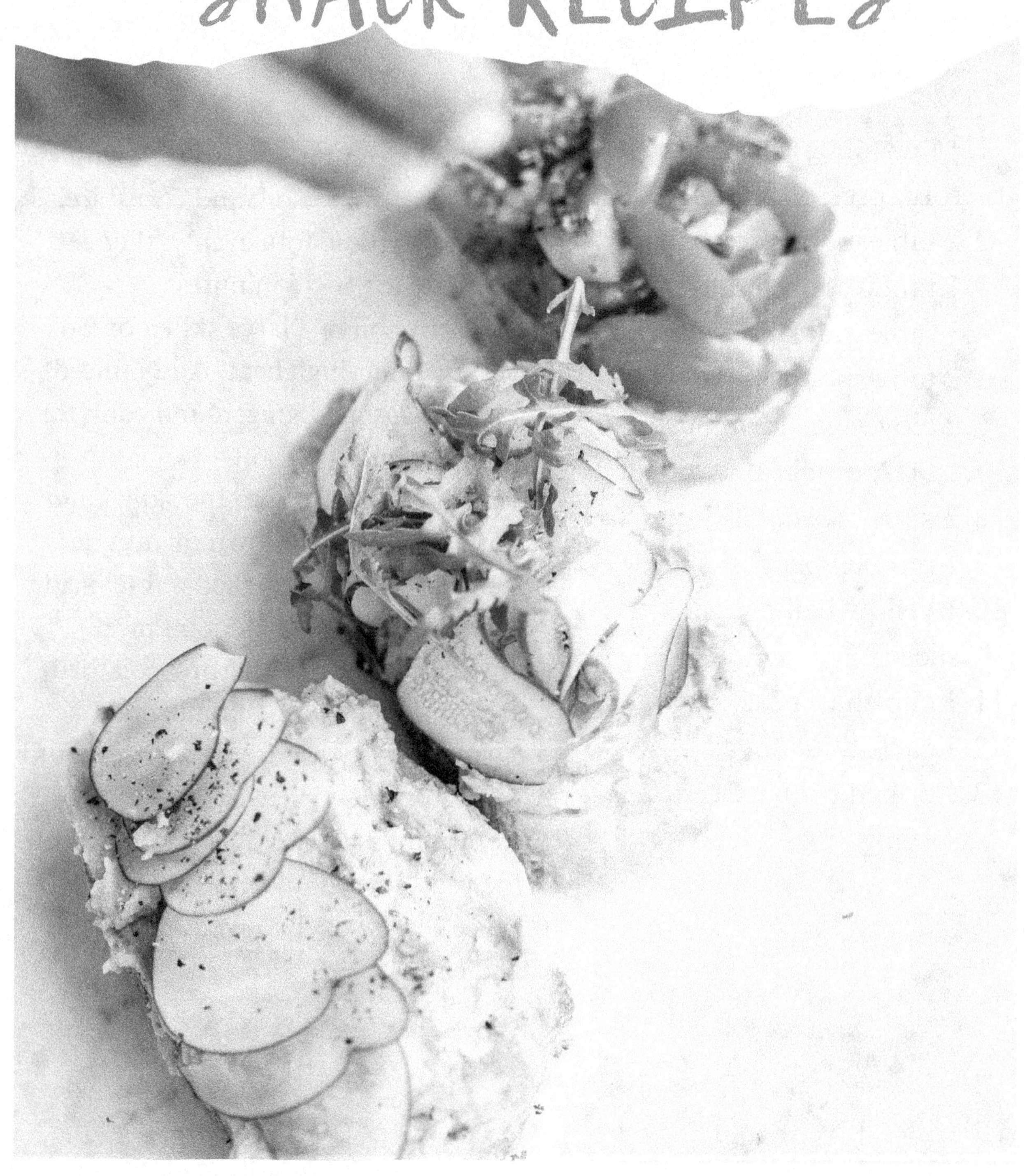

Avocado Toast with Tomato and Basil

Calories	Protein	Carbohydrates	Fiber	Fat
180	5g	20g	8g	10g

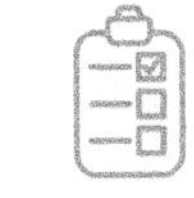

5 minutes

5 minutes

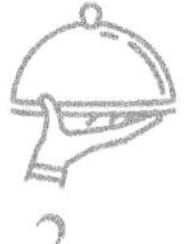

2

INGREDIENTS

1. 1 ripe avocado
2. 2 slices whole grain bread
3. 1 tomato, sliced
4. Fresh basil leaves
5. Salt and pepper to taste

INSTRUCTIONS

1. Toast the slices of bread until golden brown.
2. Mash the avocado and spread it evenly onto the toasted bread slices.
3. Top each slice with sliced tomato and fresh basil leaves.
4. Season with salt and pepper to taste.

Greek Yogurt with Berries and Almonds

Calories	Protein	Carbohydrates	Fiber	Fat
250	20g	20g	5g	12g

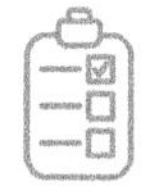

5 minutes

5 minutes

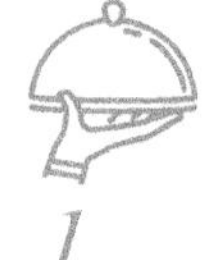

1

INGREDIENTS

1. 1 cup Greek yogurt
2. 1/2 cup mixed berries (strawberries, blueberries, raspberries)
3. 1 tablespoon almonds, chopped
4. Drizzle of honey (optional)

INSTRUCTIONS

1. Spoon Greek yogurt into a bowl.
2. Top with mixed berries and chopped almonds.
3. Drizzle with honey if desired.

Hummus and Veggie Sticks

Calories	Protein	Carbohydrates	Fiber	Fat
120	5g	12g	5g	7g

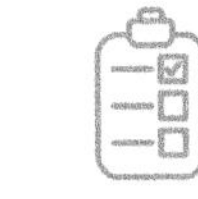 5 minutes

 0 minutes

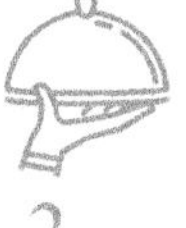 2

INGREDIENTS

1. 1/2 cup hummus
2. Carrot sticks
3. Cucumber slices
4. Bell pepper strips

INSTRUCTIONS

1. Place hummus in a small bowl.
2. Arrange carrot sticks, cucumber slices, and bell pepper strips on a plate.
3. Dip the veggie sticks into the hummus and enjoy.

Almond Butter Banana Slices

Calories	Protein	Carbohydrates	Fiber	Fat
200	5g	25g	5g	10g

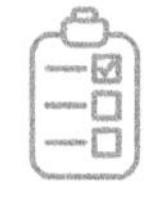 5 minutes

 0 minutes

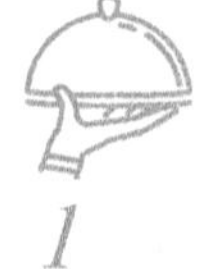 1

INGREDIENTS

1. 1 banana, sliced
2. 2 tablespoons almond butter
3. Optional toppings: chia seeds, shredded coconut, cinnamon

INSTRUCTIONS

1. Spread almond butter onto banana slices.
2. Sprinkle with optional toppings if desired.

Quinoa Salad Cups

Calories	Protein	Carbohydrates	Fiber	Fat
200	5g	25g	5g	10g

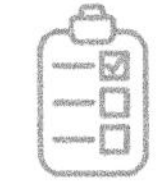 10 minutes

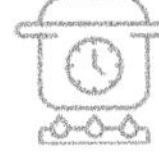 15 minutes (for cooking quinoa)

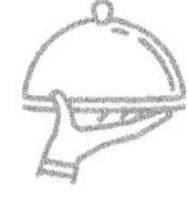 2

INGREDIENTS

1. 1 cup cooked quinoa
2. Cherry tomatoes, halved
3. Cucumber, diced
4. Red onion, finely chopped
5. Fresh parsley, chopped
6. Lemon juice
7. Olive oil
8. Salt and pepper to taste

INSTRUCTIONS

1. In a bowl, combine cooked quinoa, cherry tomatoes, cucumber, red onion, and parsley.
2. Drizzle with lemon juice and olive oil.
3. Season with salt and pepper to taste.
4. Serve the quinoa salad in small cups or lettuce leaves.

Quinoa Salad Cups

Calories	Protein	Carbohydrates	Fiber	Fat
220	6g	30g	5g	8g

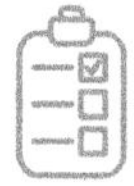 10 minutes

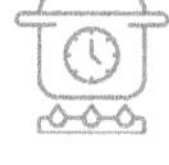 15 minutes (for cooking quinoa)

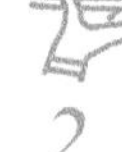 2

INGREDIENTS

1. 1 cup cooked quinoa
2. Cherry tomatoes, halved
3. Cucumber, diced
4. Red onion, finely chopped
5. Fresh parsley, chopped
6. Lemon juice
7. Olive oil
8. Salt and pepper to taste

INSTRUCTIONS

1. In a bowl, combine cooked quinoa, cherry tomatoes, cucumber, red onion, and parsley.
2. Drizzle with lemon juice and olive oil.
3. Season with salt and pepper to taste.
4. Serve the quinoa salad in small cups or lettuce leaves.

Rice Cake with Almond Butter and Banana

Calories	Protein	Carbohydrates	Fiber	Fat
150	4g	20g	3g	7g

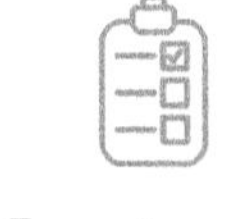 5 minutes

 0 minutes

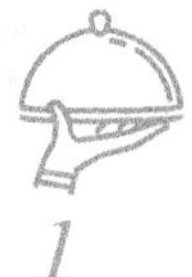 1

INGREDIENTS

1. 1 rice cake
2. 1 tablespoon almond butter
3. 1/2 banana, sliced
4. Optional toppings: honey, cinnamon

INSTRUCTIONS

1. Spread almond butter onto the rice cake.
2. Top with sliced banana.
3. Drizzle with honey and sprinkle with cinnamon if desired.

Edamame Salad

Calories	Protein	Carbohydrates	Fiber	Fat
160	9g	18g	6g	7g

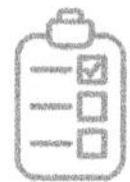 10 minutes

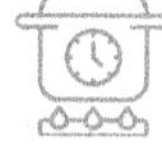 5 minutes (for cooking edamame)

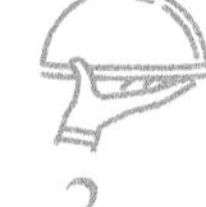 2

INGREDIENTS

1. 1 cup cooked edamame
2. Cherry tomatoes, halved
3. Red bell pepper, diced
4. Red onion, finely chopped
5. Fresh cilantro, chopped
6. Lime juice
7. Olive oil
8. Salt and pepper to taste

INSTRUCTIONS

1. In a bowl, combine cooked edamame, cherry tomatoes, red bell pepper, red onion, and cilantro.
2. Drizzle with lime juice and olive oil.
3. Season with salt and pepper to taste.

Cottage Cheese with Pineapple

Calories	Protein	Carbohydrates	Fiber	Fat
150	15g	20g	2g	2g

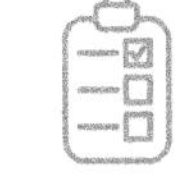 5 minutes

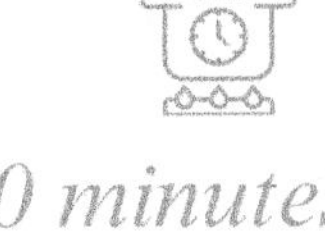 0 minutes

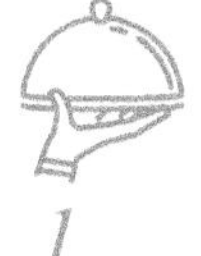 1

INGREDIENTS

1. 1/2 cup cottage cheese
2. 1/2 cup fresh pineapple chunks
3. Optional toppings: shredded coconut, chopped nuts

INSTRUCTIONS

1. Spoon cottage cheese into a bowl.
2. Top with fresh pineapple chunks.
3. Sprinkle with optional toppings if desired.

Stuffed Bell Pepper Halves

Calories	Protein	Carbohydrates	Fiber	Fat
100	3g	15g	5g	5g

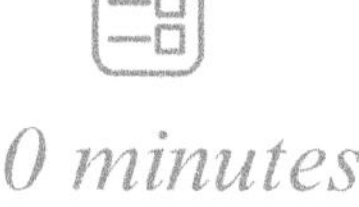 10 minutes

0 minutes

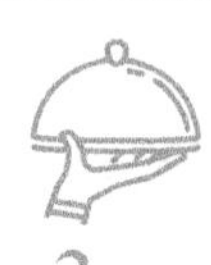 2

INGREDIENTS

1. 1 bell pepper, halved and deseeded
2. Hummus or guacamole
3. Sliced cucumber
4. Cherry tomatoes, halved
5. Sprouts or microgreens
6. Optional toppings: balsamic glaze, sesame seeds

INSTRUCTIONS

1. Fill each bell pepper half with hummus or guacamole.
2. Top with sliced cucumber, cherry tomatoes, and sprouts.
3. Drizzle with balsamic glaze and sprinkle with sesame seeds if desired.

Apple Slices with Almond Butter and Chia Seeds

Calories	Protein	Carbohydrates	Fiber	Fat
200	5g	25g	8g	10g

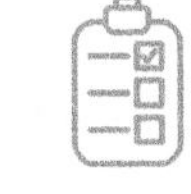 5 minutes

 0 minutes

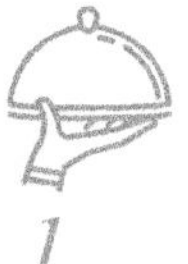 1

INGREDIENTS

1. 1 apple, sliced
2. 2 tablespoons almond butter
3. 1 tablespoon chia seeds

INSTRUCTIONS

1. Spread almond butter onto apple slices.
2. Sprinkle with chia seeds.

CHAPTER 8

DESSERT RECIPES

Berry Chia Pudding

Calories	Protein	Carbohydrates	Fiber	Fat
180	4g	24g	10g	8g

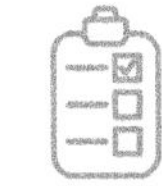 10 minutes

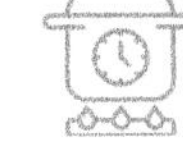 2 hours (chilling time)

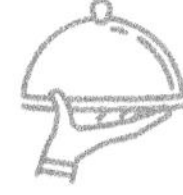 2

INGREDIENTS

1. 1/4 cup chia seeds
2. 1 cup unsweetened almond milk
3. 1/2 cup mixed berries (strawberries, blueberries, raspberries)
4. 1 tablespoon honey or maple syrup (optional)

INSTRUCTIONS

1. In a bowl, combine chia seeds and almond milk. Stir well and let it sit for 10 minutes.
2. Stir the mixture again to prevent clumping. Refrigerate for at least 2 hours or overnight.
3. Before serving, top the pudding with mixed berries and drizzle with honey or maple syrup if desired.

Baked Apples with Cinnamon

Calories	Protein	Carbohydrates	Fiber	Fat
150	1g	38g	6g	1g

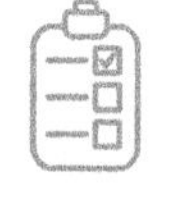 *10 minutes*

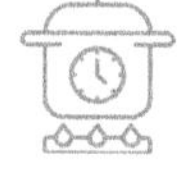 *25-30 minutes*

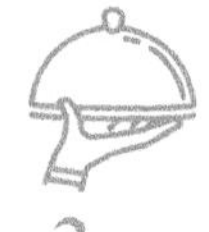 *2*

INGREDIENTS

1. 2 apples (Granny Smith or Fuji)
2. 1 teaspoon cinnamon
3. 1 tablespoon honey or maple syrup
4. 1/4 cup chopped walnuts (optional)

INSTRUCTIONS

1. Preheat the oven to 375°F (190°C).
2. Core the apples and place them in a baking dish.
3. Sprinkle cinnamon over the apples and drizzle with honey or maple syrup.
4. Bake for 25-30 minutes until apples are tender.
5. Serve warm, topped with chopped walnuts if desired.

Banana Oat Cookies

Calories	Protein	Carbohydrates	Fiber	Fat
80	2g	12g	2g	3g

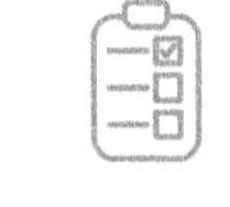 10 minutes

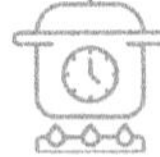 15-20 minutes

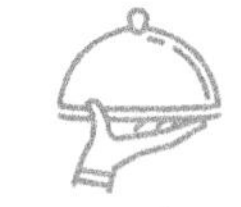 12 cookies

INGREDIENTS

1. 2 ripe bananas, mashed
2. 1 cup rolled oats
3. 1/4 cup chopped nuts (walnuts or almonds)
4. 1/4 cup dark chocolate chips (optional)
5. 1 teaspoon vanilla extract
6. 1/2 teaspoon cinnamon

INSTRUCTIONS

1. Preheat the oven to 350°F (175°C) and line a baking sheet with parchment paper.
2. In a bowl, combine mashed bananas, rolled oats, chopped nuts, chocolate chips (if using), vanilla extract, and cinnamon. Mix until well combined.
3. Drop spoonfuls of the mixture onto the prepared baking sheet, spacing them apart.
4. Bake for 15-20 minutes until golden brown.
5. Allow cookies to cool before serving.

Coconut Mango Sorbet

Calories	Protein	Carbohydrates	Fiber	Fat
120	1g	20g	2g	5g

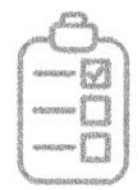

5 minutes

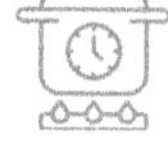

2-3 hours (freezing time)

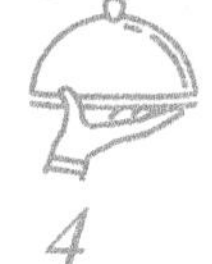

4

INGREDIENTS

1. 2 cups frozen mango chunks
2. 1/2 cup coconut milk
3. 1 tablespoon honey or maple syrup (optional)
4. 1 teaspoon lime juice

INSTRUCTIONS

1. In a blender, combine frozen mango chunks, coconut milk, honey or maple syrup (if using), and lime juice. Blend until smooth and creamy.
2. Transfer the mixture to a shallow dish and freeze for 2-3 hours, stirring occasionally.
3. Once set, scoop the sorbet into bowls and serve immediately.

Almond Butter Date Balls

Calories	Protein	Carbohydrates	Fiber	Fat
110	2g	12g	2g	6g

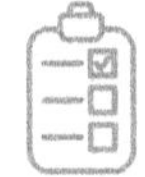

15 minutes

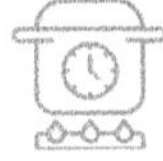

30 minutes (chilling time)

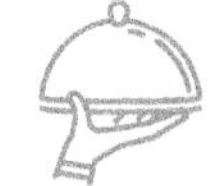

12 balls

INGREDIENTS

1. 1 cup pitted dates
2. 1/2 cup almond butter
3. 1/4 cup almond flour
4. 1/4 cup shredded coconut (unsweetened)
5. 1 teaspoon vanilla extract
6. Pinch of sea salt

INSTRUCTIONS

1. In a food processor, combine pitted dates, almond butter, almond flour, shredded coconut, vanilla extract, and a pinch of sea salt. Pulse until the mixture forms a sticky dough.
2. Roll the dough into small balls using your hands.
3. Roll the balls in additional shredded coconut if desired.
4. Refrigerate for at least 30 minutes before serving.

Blueberry Oat Bars

Calories	Protein	Carbohydrates	Fiber	Fat
180	4g	28g	4g	6g

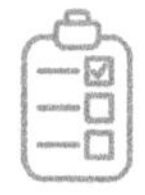 10 minutes

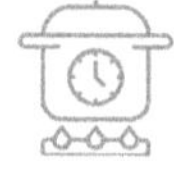 25-30 minutes

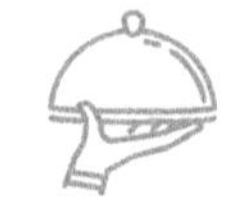 8 bars

INGREDIENTS

1. 2 cups rolled oats
2. 1 cup blueberries (fresh or frozen)
3. 1/4 cup maple syrup
4. 1/4 cup almond butter
5. 1/4 cup almond milk
6. 1 teaspoon vanilla extract
7. Pinch of sea salt

INSTRUCTIONS

1. Preheat the oven to 350°F (175°C) and line a baking dish with parchment paper.
2. In a bowl, mix together rolled oats, blueberries, maple syrup, almond butter, almond milk, vanilla extract, and a pinch of sea salt until well combined.
3. Press the mixture evenly into the prepared baking dish.
4. Bake for 25-30 minutes until golden brown.
5. Allow to cool before slicing into bars.

Chocolate Avocado Mousse

Calories	Protein	Carbohydrates	Fiber	Fat
180	3g	18g	7g	12g

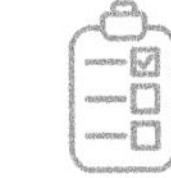

10 minutes

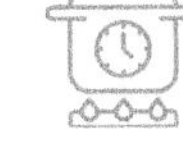

30 minutes (chilling time)

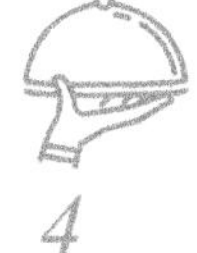

4

INGREDIENTS

1. 2 ripe avocados
2. 1/4 cup cocoa powder (unsweetened)
3. 1/4 cup honey or maple syrup
4. 1 teaspoon vanilla extract
5. Pinch of sea salt
6. Fresh berries for serving (optional)

INSTRUCTIONS

1. In a food processor or blender, combine ripe avocados, cocoa powder, honey or maple syrup, vanilla extract, and a pinch of sea salt. Blend until smooth and creamy.
2. Transfer the mousse to serving bowls or glasses.
3. Refrigerate for at least 30 minutes before serving.
4. Serve topped with fresh berries if desired.

Peanut Butter Banana Nice Cream

Calories	Protein	Carbohydrates	Fiber	Fat
200	4g	27g	4g	9g

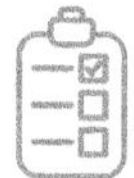

5 minutes

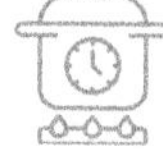

1-2 hours (freezing time, optional)

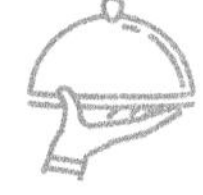

2

INGREDIENTS

1. 2 ripe bananas, sliced and frozen
2. 2 tablespoons peanut butter (or almond butter)
3. 1/4 cup unsweetened almond milk
4. 1 teaspoon vanilla extract
5. 1 tablespoon dark chocolate chips (optional)

INSTRUCTIONS

1. In a blender or food processor, combine frozen banana slices, peanut butter, almond milk, and vanilla extract. Blend until smooth and creamy.
2. Transfer the nice cream to a bowl and fold in dark chocolate chips if desired.
3. Serve immediately as soft-serve ice cream or freeze for 1-2 hours for a firmer texture.

Lemon Poppy Seed Muffins

Calories	Protein	Carbohydrates	Fiber	Fat
180	5g	14g	3g	12g

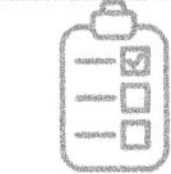 10 minutes

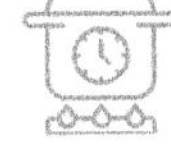 20-25 minutes

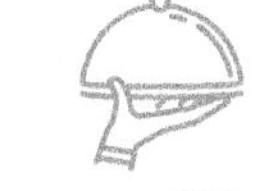 12 muffins

INGREDIENTS

1. 1 1/2 cups almond flour
2. 1/4 cup coconut flour
3. 1/4 cup honey or maple syrup
4. 1/4 cup melted coconut oil
5. 3 eggs
6. 1/4 cup fresh lemon juice
7. Zest of 1 lemon
8. 1 tablespoon poppy seeds
9. 1 teaspoon baking soda
10. Pinch of sea salt

INSTRUCTIONS

1. Preheat the oven to 350°F (175°C) and line a muffin tin with paper liners.
2. In a bowl, whisk together almond flour, coconut flour, honey or maple syrup, melted coconut oil, eggs, lemon juice, lemon zest, poppy seeds, baking soda, and a pinch of sea salt until smooth.
3. Divide the batter evenly among the muffin cups.
4. Bake for 20-25 minutes until golden brown and a toothpick inserted into the center comes out clean.
5. Allow muffins to cool before serving.

Peach Cobbler with Almond Flour Topping

Calories	Protein	Carbohydrates	Fiber	Fat
220	4g	28g	5g	12g

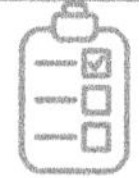 15 minutes

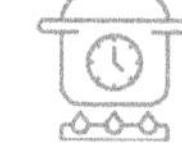 25-30 minutes

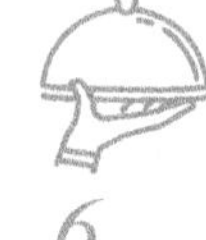 6

INGREDIENTS

1. 4 cups sliced peaches (fresh or frozen)
2. 1 tablespoon honey or maple syrup
3. 1 teaspoon cinnamon
4. 1/2 cup almond flour
5. 1/4 cup chopped almonds
6. 2 tablespoons coconut oil (solid)
7. 2 tablespoons honey or maple syrup
8. 1 teaspoon vanilla extract
9. Pinch of sea salt

INSTRUCTIONS

1. Preheat the oven to 350°F (175°C) and lightly grease a baking dish.
2. In a bowl, toss sliced peaches with honey or maple syrup and cinnamon. Transfer to the prepared baking dish.
3. In another bowl, combine almond flour, chopped almonds, coconut oil, honey or maple syrup, vanilla extract, and a pinch of sea salt. Mix until crumbly.
4. Spread the almond flour topping evenly over the peaches.
5. Bake for 25-30 minutes until the topping is golden brown and the peaches are bubbling.
6. Allow to cool slightly before serving.

CHAPTER 9
BEVERAGES

Green Smoothie

Calories	Protein	Carbohydrates	Fiber	Fat
130	3g	29g	5g	2g

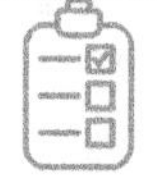 *5 minutes*

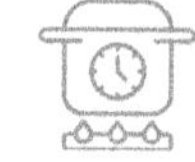 *5 minutes*

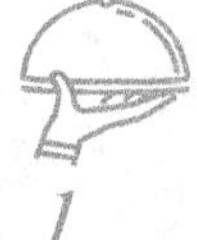 *1*

INGREDIENTS

1. 1 cup spinach
2. 1/2 cup cucumber, peeled and chopped
3. 1/2 banana
4. 1/2 cup pineapple chunks
5. 1/2 cup almond milk

INSTRUCTIONS

1. Add all ingredients to a blender.
2. Blend until smooth and creamy.
3. Serve immediately and enjoy!

Turmeric Latte

Calories	Protein	Carbohydrates	Fiber	Fat
60	1g	9g	1g	3g

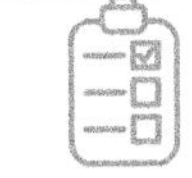 2 minutes

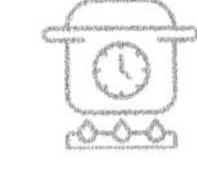 5 minutes

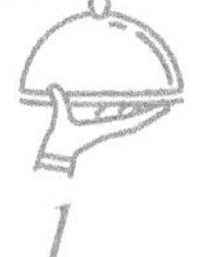 1

INGREDIENTS

1. 1 cup almond milk
2. 1 teaspoon ground turmeric
3. 1/2 teaspoon ground cinnamon
4. 1/4 teaspoon ground ginger
5. 1 teaspoon honey (optional)

INSTRUCTIONS

1. In a small saucepan, heat almond milk over medium heat until warm but not boiling.
2. Whisk in ground turmeric, cinnamon, and ginger until well combined.
3. Stir in honey if desired.
4. Pour into a mug and serve hot.

Berry Beet Smoothie1

Calories	Protein	Carbohydrates	Fiber	Fat
150	8g	27g	5g	2g

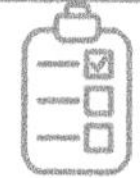 3 minutes

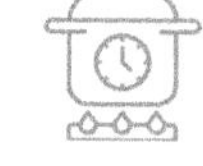 5 minutes

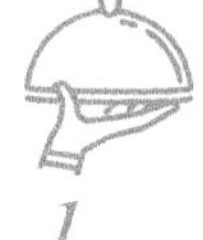 1

INGREDIENTS

1. 1/2 cup mixed berries (such as strawberries, blueberries, raspberries)
2. 1/2 small beet, peeled and chopped
3. 1/2 cup Greek yogurt
4. 1/4 cup almond milk
5. 1 tablespoon honey (optional)

INSTRUCTIONS

1. Combine all ingredients in a blender.
2. Blend until smooth and creamy.
3. Taste and add honey if desired for sweetness.
4. Pour into a glass and enjoy!

Matcha Green Tea Latte

Calories	Protein	Carbohydrates	Fiber	Fat
60	1g	9g	1g	3g

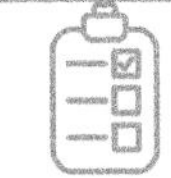 2 minutes

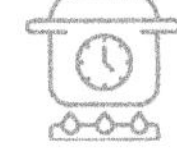 5 minutes

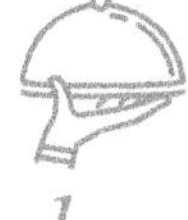 1

INGREDIENTS

1. 1 teaspoon matcha green tea powder
2. 1 cup almond milk
3. 1 teaspoon honey (optional)

INSTRUCTIONS

1. Heat almond milk in a small saucepan over medium heat until warm but not boiling.
2. In a mug, whisk together matcha green tea powder and a small amount of hot water to form a paste.
3. Pour warm almond milk over the matcha paste and whisk until frothy.
4. Sweeten with honey if desired.
5. Serve hot and enjoy!

Chia Seed Smoothie

Calories	Protein	Carbohydrates	Fiber	Fat
150	5g	28g	10g	4g

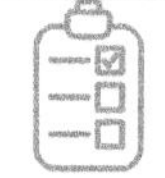

10 minutes (including soaking chia seeds)

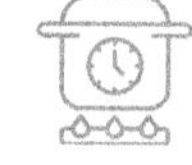

5 minutes

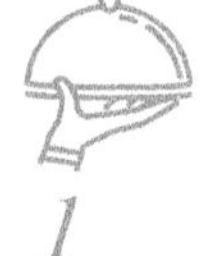

1

INGREDIENTS

1. 1 tablespoon chia seeds
2. 1/2 cup mixed berries
3. 1/2 banana
4. 1/2 cup spinach
5. 1/2 cup coconut water

INSTRUCTIONS

1. In a glass or jar, combine chia seeds and coconut water. Let sit for 5-10 minutes until chia seeds swell and form a gel-like consistency.
2. In a blender, combine soaked chia seeds, mixed berries, banana, and spinach.
3. Blend until smooth and creamy.
4. Pour into a glass and serve immediately.

Ginger Lemonade

Calories	Protein	Carbohydrates	Fiber	Fat
70	0g	19g	0g	0g

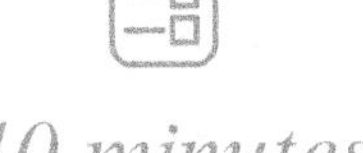

10 minutes   *5 minutes*   *2*

INGREDIENTS

1. 1 tablespoon freshly grated ginger
2. 2 tablespoons honey
3. 1/4 cup fresh lemon juice
4. 2 cups water
5. Ice cubes

INSTRUCTIONS

1. In a small saucepan, combine grated ginger, honey, and water.
2. Heat over medium heat until honey is dissolved and ginger is fragrant, about 5 minutes.
3. Remove from heat and let cool to room temperature.
4. Strain the ginger-infused liquid into a pitcher.
5. Stir in fresh lemon juice and add ice cubes.
6. Serve chilled and enjoy!

Cucumber Mint Infused Water

Calories	Protein	Carbohydrates	Fiber	Fat
0	0g	0g	0g	0g

5 minutes | 1 minute | 4

INGREDIENTS

1. 1/2 cucumber, thinly sliced
2. 1/4 cup fresh mint leaves
3. 4 cups water
4. Ice cubes

INSTRUCTIONS

1. In a pitcher, combine cucumber slices and fresh mint leaves.
2. Fill the pitcher with water and stir to combine.
3. Refrigerate for at least 1 hour to allow the flavors to infuse.
4. Serve chilled over ice cubes.

Pineapple Ginger Smoothie

Calories	Protein	Carbohydrates	Fiber	Fat
170	7g	33g	3g	2g

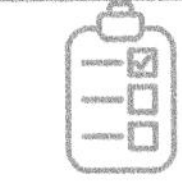 3 minutes

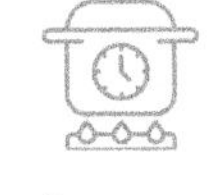 5 minutes

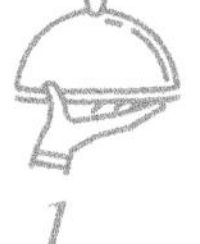 1

INGREDIENTS

1. 1 cup fresh pineapple chunks
2. 1/2 inch piece of ginger, peeled
3. 1/2 cup Greek yogurt
4. 1/4 cup almond milk
5. 1 tablespoon honey (optional)

INSTRUCTIONS

1. Combine all ingredients in a blender.
2. Blend until smooth and creamy.
3. Taste and add honey if desired for sweetness.
4. Pour into a glass and serve immediately.

Berry Basil Infused Water

Calories	Protein	Carbohydrates	Fiber	Fat
0	0g	0g	0g	0g

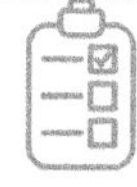 5 minutes

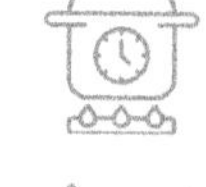 1 minute

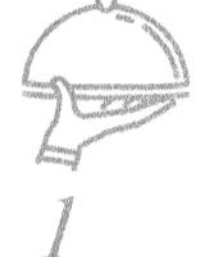 1

INGREDIENTS

1. 1/2 cup mixed berries (such as strawberries, blueberries, raspberries)
2. 1/4 cup fresh basil leaves
3. 4 cups water
4. Ice cubes

INSTRUCTIONS

1. In a pitcher, combine mixed berries and fresh basil leaves.
2. Fill the pitcher with water and stir to combine.
3. Refrigerate for at least 1 hour to allow the flavors to infuse.
4. Serve chilled over ice cubes.

Coconut Watermelon Cooler

Calories	Protein	Carbohydrates	Fiber	Fat
70	1g	17g	1g	0g

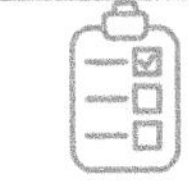 3 minutes

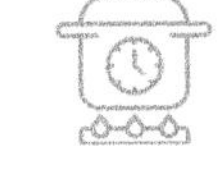 5 minutes

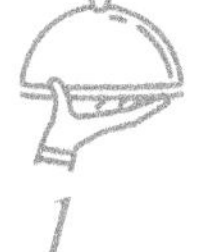 1

INGREDIENTS

1. 1 cup fresh watermelon chunks
2. 1/2 cup coconut water
3. 1 tablespoon fresh lime juice
4. Ice cubes

INSTRUCTIONS

1. In a blender, combine watermelon chunks, coconut water, and fresh lime juice.
2. Blend until smooth and well combined.
3. Taste and adjust sweetness or acidity if desired.
4. Serve chilled over ice cubes.

Coconut Watermelon Cooler

Calories	Protein	Carbohydrates	Fiber	Fat
70	1g	17g	1g	0g

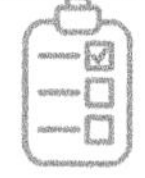 3 minutes

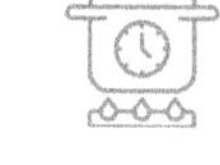 5 minutes

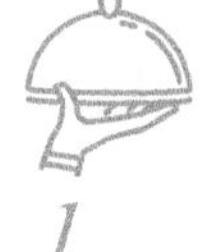 1

INGREDIENTS

1. 1 cup fresh watermelon chunks
2. 1/2 cup coconut water
3. 1 tablespoon fresh lime juice
4. Ice cubes

INSTRUCTIONS

1. In a blender, combine watermelon chunks, coconut water, and fresh lime juice.
2. Blend until smooth and well combined.
3. Taste and adjust sweetness or acidity if desired.
4. Serve chilled over ice cubes.

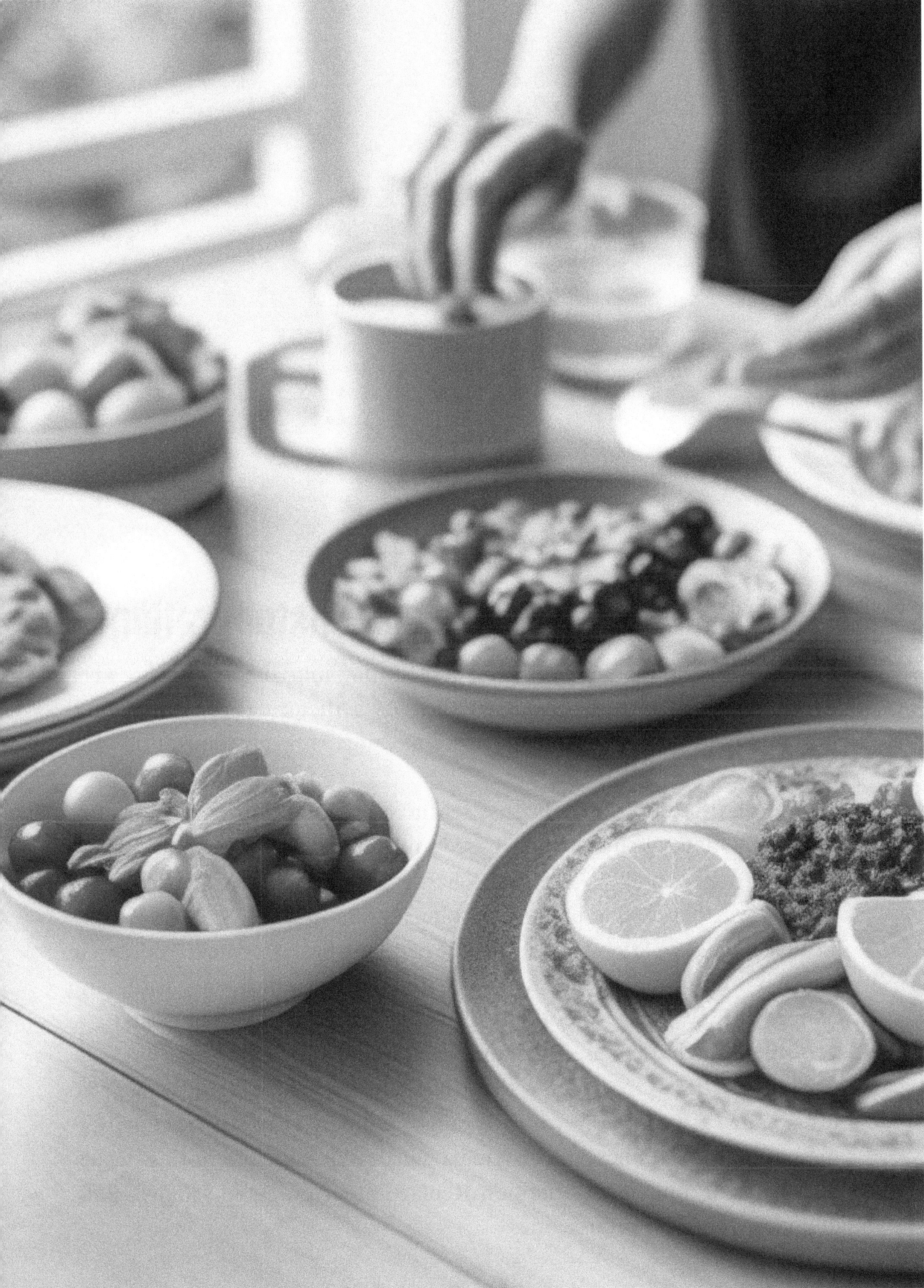

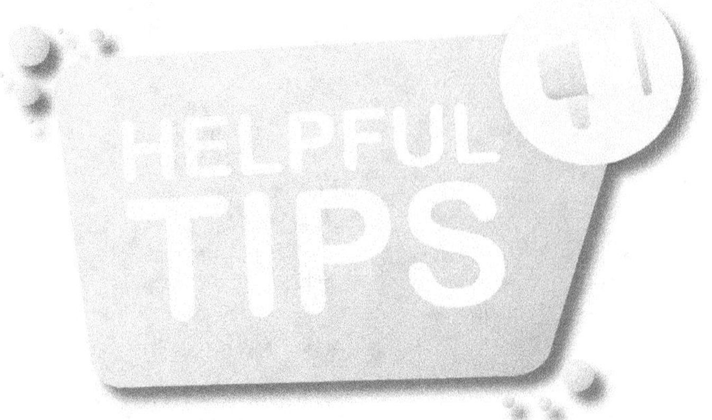

CHAPTER 10

Tips for Substitutions and Customization

For Type A dieters, modifying and substituting ingredients in recipes is a terrific method to make meals fit their own dietary requirements and tastes. The following are some useful hints for customization and substitutions:

Dairy Substitutes: If you're lactose sensitive or would rather not consume dairy, you may substitute plant-based milks like almond, coconut, or soy milk for cow's milk in recipes. These substitutes don't lose taste or texture, whether used in baking, cooking, or smoothies.

Protein Sources: Try using a variety of plant-based protein sources in place of meat in dishes, such as lentils, beans, chickpeas, tofu, and tempeh. These high-protein substitutes provide vital nutrients and are versatile enough to be used in soups, salads, and stir-fries.

Grain Varieties: Go beyond the usual choices of rice and wheat to investigate a range of whole grains. Quinoa, brown rice, barley, buckwheat, and millet are all great substitutes with interesting tastes, textures, and nutritional qualities. Replace other grains in salads, pilafs, and grain bowls with these ones.

Gluten-Free Options: There are many gluten-free options available for those who follow a gluten-free diet, including brown rice noodles, quinoa pasta, and flour blends. These substitutes may be used in recipes for baked goods, bread, and pasta meals instead of wheat-based items.

Sweeteners: When sweetening dishes, think about using natural sweeteners like honey, maple syrup, or coconut sugar in place of refined sugars. These substitutes provide more sweetness, along with more antioxidants and minerals. When using sweeteners, pay attention to portion amounts and adjust according to taste.

Herbs & Spices: To add flavor to your food without using a lot of salt or harmful seasonings, try experimenting with different herbs and spices. While spices like turmeric, ginger, cinnamon, and cumin may give savory foods more depth and complexity, fresh herbs like basil, parsley, cilantro, and mint can improve the flavor of salads, soups, and sauces.

Healthy Fats: Instead of saturated and trans fats in recipes, use healthy fat sources such as avocado, olive oil, nuts, and seeds. These fats may be utilized in baking, cooking, and salad dressings and provide vital fatty acids that promote heart health.

Portion Control: Be mindful of serving sizes and attentive to your body's signals of hunger and fullness. Savor each mouthful and practice mindful eating to prevent overindulging. Adapt serving sizes to your own energy requirements and degree of exercise.

Hydration: Throughout the day, make sure you drink plenty of water to stay hydrated. In addition to being beneficial for promoting digestion and preventing overeating, hydration is crucial for general health and well-being. For more taste and hydration, try adding cucumbers, fresh fruits, or herbs to the water.

Last but not least, pay attention to your body and respect its distinct requirements and preferences. Observe your reactions to various meals and modify your diet appropriately. Keep in mind that each individual has a unique physique, so what suits one may not suit another.

By may make tasty and nutritious meals that complement your Type A blood type and promote your general health and well-being by using these replacement and modification guidelines when you plan and prepare your meals. Try a variety of ingredients, tastes, and cooking methods to see what suits you the best.

Adjusting Recipes to Fit Individual Tastes

One great technique for Type A dieters to customize their meals and make sure they love what they eat while still following their dietary rules is to modify recipes to suit individual preferences. Here's how to modify recipes to fit personal tastes:

Flavor Profiles: To improve the flavor of food, try experimenting with various herbs, spices, and seasonings. If a recipe asks for an ingredient you don't like, consider using a taste you do like instead. Try substituting parsley or basil for cilantro, for instance, if a recipe asks for it but you don't like the flavor.

Texture Preferences: When cooking, take into account your guests' preferences for texture. Make the necessary adjustments to ingredients or cooking techniques if you want your food to be more crunchy or creamy. Consider mixing only a part of the soup and leaving the remainder unblended, for example, if a soup recipe calls for blending all the ingredients but you prefer a chunkier texture.

Sweetness Level: You may vary the quantity of sweeteners used in recipes to make them as sweet as you want. If a recipe specifies a certain quantity of honey or sugar and you'd like it to be less sweet, consider using natural substitutes like maple syrup or pureed fruit.

Sweet vs. Savory: Some people have a preference for sweet tastes over savory ones. Add extra savory ingredients, such as garlic, onions, or spices, to balance out a meal that you perceive to be excessively sweet. On the other hand, if a meal seems too salty, think about including some sweetness with dried fruit or honey.

Substituting items to better fit your nutritional needs or taste preferences is nothing to be frightened of. Feel free to substitute tofu for chicken, for instance, if a recipe calls for it but you prefer the protein. Similarly, if a recipe calls for an item that you dislike or are allergic to, substitute something that suits your preferences.

Portion Sizes: Modify serving sizes in accordance with your energy requirements and appetite. To prevent leftovers, cut the ingredients in half if a dish calls for four people but you're only cooking for two. Alternatively, you may scale up the recipe to make sure you have enough food to satiate your appetite if you like bigger servings.

Cooking Methods: Experiment with various cooking methods to get the outcomes you want. Whatever your favorite cooking method—grilling, sautéing, baking, or steaming—make sure to modify recipes to suit it. Try out several techniques to see which ones give you the desired taste and texture.

Garnishes and toppers: Use inventive garnishes and toppers to enhance the taste and appearance of food. To improve the overall appearance and flavor of your dishes, add fresh herbs, citrus zest, nuts, seeds, or a drizzle of sauce. Tailor garnishes to your dish's tastes and add a unique touch to your culinary masterpieces.

Type A dieters may prepare meals that are not only wholesome and gratifying but also pleasurable by tailoring recipes to suit personal preferences. In order to customize recipes to your particular tastes and dietary requirements, don't be afraid to be creative in the kitchen and experiment with various ingredients, flavors, and cooking methods.

CHAPTER 11

Meal Planning and Prepping

For Type A dieters to keep on track with their dietary objectives and maintain a healthy lifestyle, meal planning and preparation are crucial habits. This is a how-to for organizing and preparing meals:

Establish Goals

To begin, decide on specific, attainable objectives for your efforts in meal planning and preparation. Take into account things like your schedule, finances, nutritional requirements, and food preferences. Ascertain how many meals you will need to prepare each day and if you will be feeding other people or yourself.

Make a Weekly Plan

Make a plan that consists of breakfast, lunch, supper, and snacks to help you organize your meals for the next week. Consider the suggestions specific to your blood type and strive to balance your meals with adequate amounts of fiber, protein, carbs, and healthy fats. To make sure you get a variety of nutrients, think about including a selection of foods.

Sun	Mon	Tue	Wed	Thu	Fri	Sat

CREATE A SHOPPING LIST.

Following your meal planning, jot down a list of every ingredient you'll need for the next week. Make sure you o1nly buy what you need by taking a look in your pantry and refrigerator to see what you already have. Adhere to your list to prevent impulsive purchases and wasteful expenditures.

PREPARE ITEMS

To make dinner preparation simpler during the week, set aside some time to prepare items ahead of time. Prepare grains or legumes in advance, wash and cut veggies, and marinate proteins. For easy access, store prepared items in the refrigerator in airtight, resealable bags or containers.

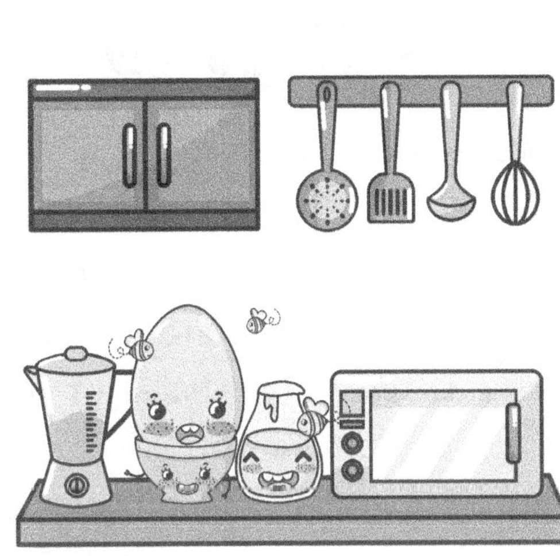

PREPARING IN BULK

Take into consideration preparing huge amounts of meals or ingredients in bulk so that they may be portioned out and enjoyed all week long. Make large batches of grains, proteins, and soups, then portion them out into individual meals that can be reheated as required. You may always have wholesome meals available and save time by preparing in bulk.

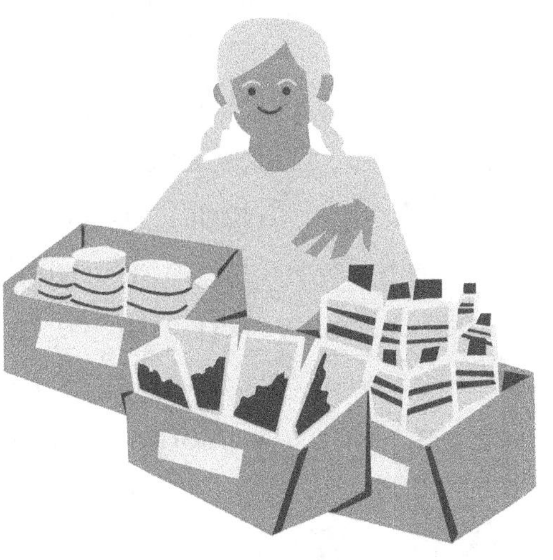

PORTION CONTROL

Make sure you're consuming the appropriate quantity of food to support your wellness and health objectives by using portion control. To portion food into sensible portions, use portion-sized containers or use scales and measuring cups. Divide up snacks and prepared components so you can get them quickly.

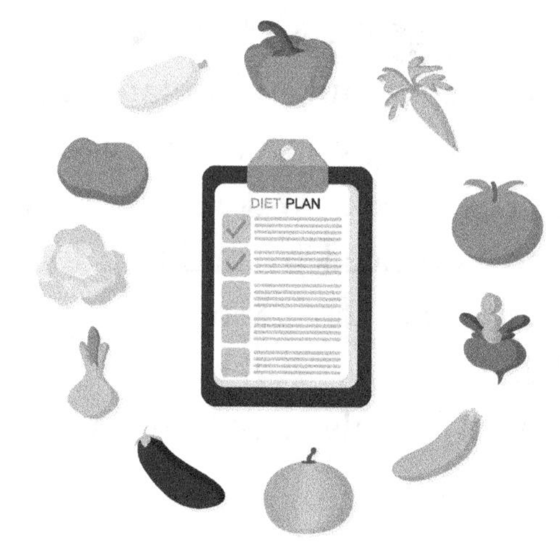

STORE CORRECTLY

Keeping your prepared meals and ingredients fresh and high-quality requires careful storage. Store prepared items in the refrigerator or freezer using airtight resealable bags or containers. Mark containers with the contents and date so you can remember what's inside and when it was made.

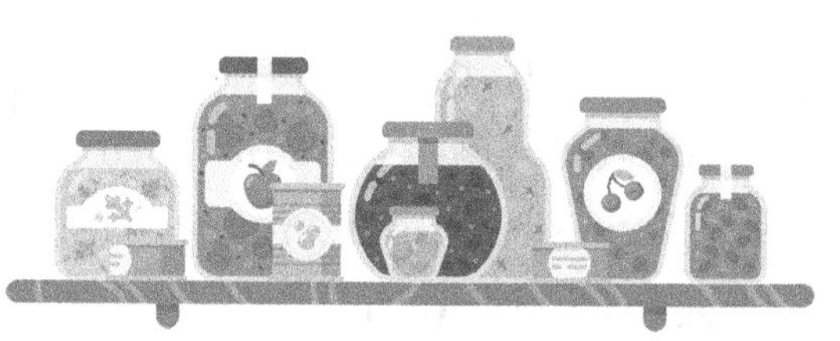

REMAIN ORGANIZED

To make food preparation and planning easier, keep your kitchen neat and orderly. Assign distinct spaces for meal preparation, storage, and cooking tools to facilitate easy retrieval of necessary items. As you go, tidy up to reduce clutter and increase productivity.

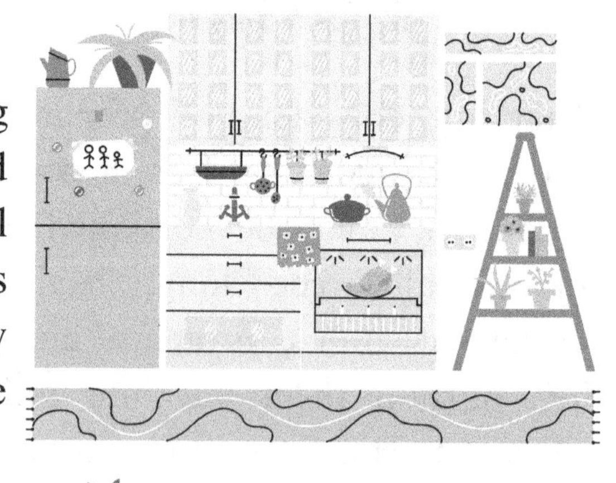

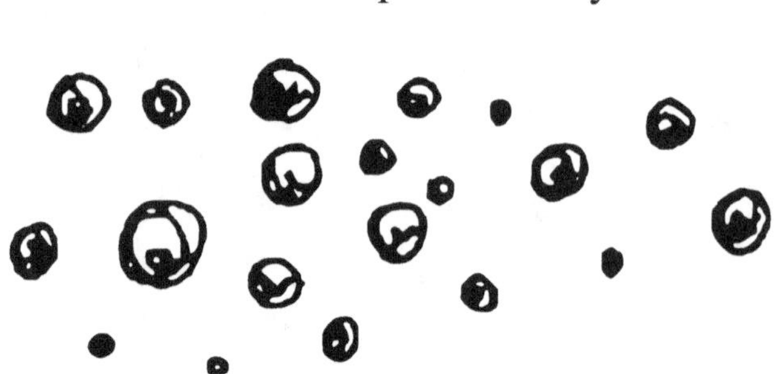

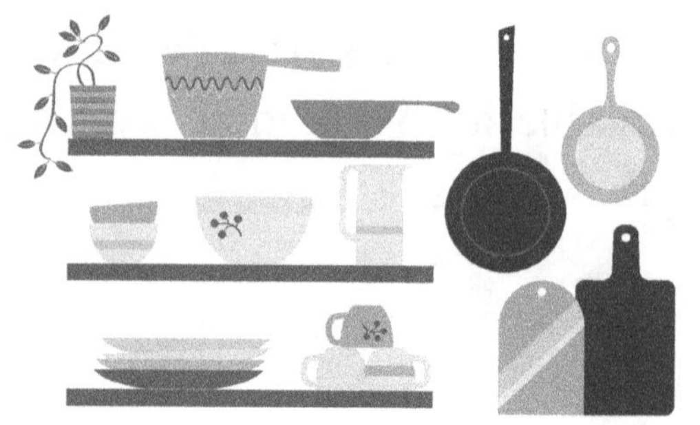

REMAIN ADAPTABLE

Modify your meal preparation and planning strategy to suit any changes in your schedule or tastes. Never be hesitant to experiment with different recipes, new ingredients, and portion proportions. Pay attention to your body's demands and modify your eating plan appropriately.

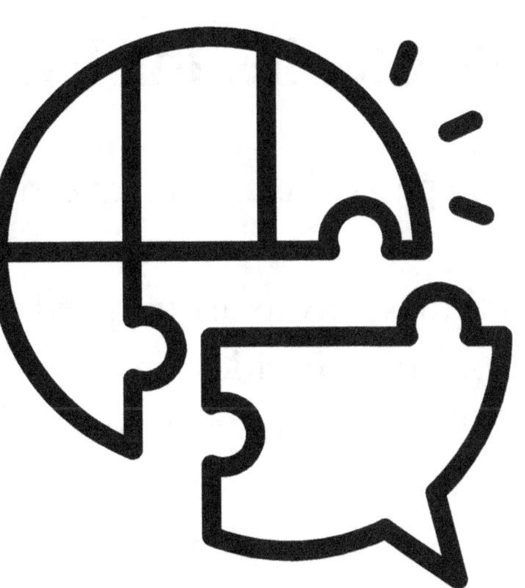

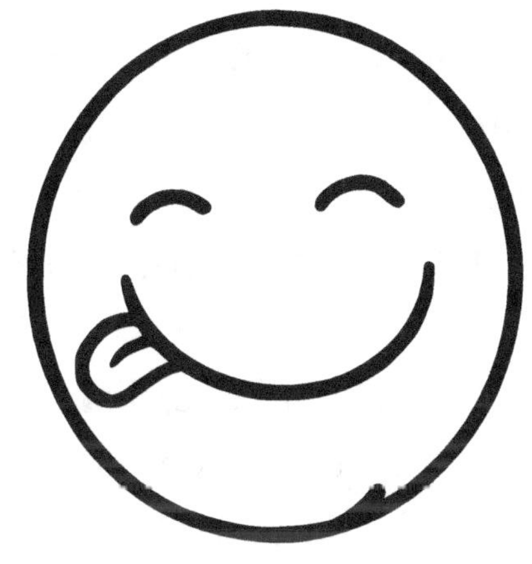

SAVOR THE BENEFITS

Savor the time-saving, stress-relieving, and health-promoting advantages of meal planning and preparation. You'll put yourself in the best possible position to succeed, adhere to your Type A diet, and reach your health objectives if you take the time to plan and prepare your meals in advance.

By can make eating healthily easier and guarantee that nourishing meals are always available by implementing meal planning and preparation into your daily routine. As a Type A dieter, you may enjoy tasty and fulfilling meals that promote your health and well-being with a little bit of planning and preparation.

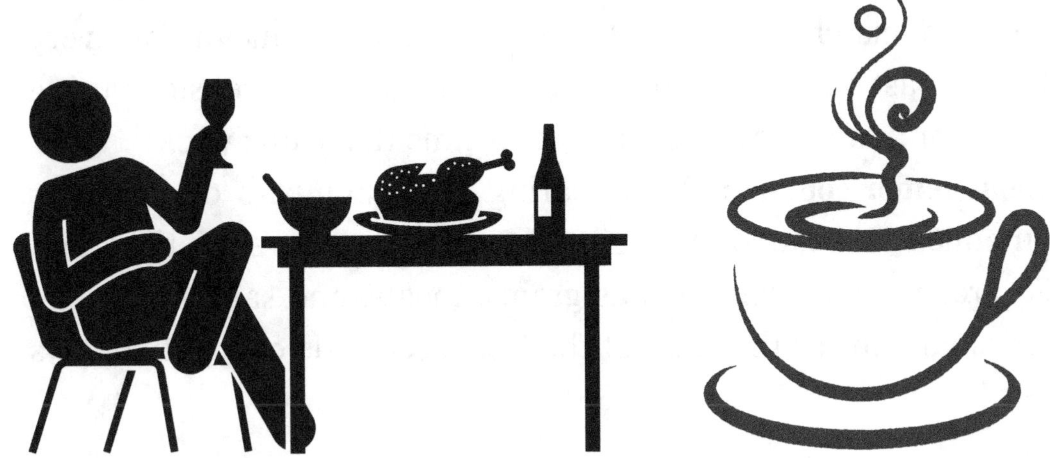

Strategies for Efficient Meal Planning

For Type A dieters to save time, minimize stress, and maintain their dietary objectives, effective meal planning is essential. The following techniques may assist in speeding up the meal planning process:

Establish a Specific Time: Allocate a particular period of time every week for the purpose of organizing meals. This may happen on a calm weeknight or on a weekend morning. It's important to be consistent, so be sure to arrange your meals at the appointed hour to make it a regular practice.

Make Use of a Meal Planning Template: Plan your meals for the next week by using a meal planning template or planner. This might be an app for meal planning, a downloadable meal planner, or a straightforward spreadsheet. You may remain focused and organized when preparing by using an ordered framework.

Take Stock: Before organizing your weekly menu, make a list of everything you have in your pantry, refrigerator, and freezer. To reduce food waste and save money, make a list of all the foods you currently have and include them in your meal plan.

Plan Around Staples: List the basic components—such as grains, meats, and vegetables—that you often utilize in your cuisine. To make grocery shopping and meal preparation easier, build your weekly menu around these essentials and use them for many meals.

Mix & Match Recipes: To produce a range of meals with comparable items, mix and match recipes rather than creating a menu for every meal. If you roast veggies for one dinner, for instance, consider using the leftovers for a salad or stir-fry at a later time that same week.

Think about batch cooking: By preparing large numbers of meals or meal components ahead of time, batch cooking may save time and work. To prepare essentials such as grains, meats, and sauces that can be used for many meals throughout the week, set aside one or two days each week.

Keep It Simple: Give priority to easy-to-follow recipes that call for few ingredients and little time to prepare. Pick meals that can be prepared in 30 minutes or less, and expedite the cooking process by using tricks like canned beans or pre-cut veggies.

Prepare for Leftovers: Make a conscious effort to make extra portions to have for lunch or supper later in the week. This will help you embrace leftovers as a time-saving tactic. Use leftovers to create new meals by mixing them with fresh ingredients or putting them in grain bowls, salads, or wraps.

Remain Adaptable: Be adaptable with your meal plan, ready to make necessary adjustments in response to scheduling or personal preference changes. Have a fallback plan, such as simple, low-preparation meals, for hectic days or unforeseen circumstances.

Evaluate and Consider: At the conclusion of every week, go over your meal plan and consider the things that went well and the things that might be done better. Utilize these suggestions to improve your meal planning procedure and make changes for the next week.

Type A dieters may lower their stress levels, save time, and make it easier to eat tasty and healthy meals all week long by putting these effective meal planning techniques into practice. You may enjoy substantial meals that promote your health and well-being without compromising convenience or taste by carefully planning and preparing them.

Batch Cooking and Freezing Tips

Freezing and batch cooking are great techniques for Type A dieters to cut down on food waste, save time, and guarantee that they always have wholesome meals available. Here are some pointers for freezing and bulk cooking:

Organize Your Cooking Sessions in Bulk: Allocate a certain period every week or month for cooking in bulk. Select the recipes you want to make in large quantities and schedule a time when you have a few hours to spare. Take into consideration meals that are simple to reheat and freeze.

Select freezer-friendly dishes: Go for dishes like soups, stews, casseroles, and sauces that can be frozen. After being frozen and then reheated, these recipes often have a better taste and texture. Steer clear of recipes calling for items that don't freeze well, such as fresh veggies with a lot of water.

Invest in High-Quality Containers: To store dishes that have been batch-cooked, spend money on freezer-safe containers or resealable bags. To maintain the freshness and safety of your food, choose sturdy, airtight, and BPA-free containers. For simple reheating, think about using portion-sized containers.

Label Everything: Write the dish's name and the preparation date on the label of each container. This makes it easier for you to keep track of the contents and expiration date of your freezer. Labeling is made simple using freezer labels, masking tape, and a permanent pen.

Cool Meals Total: Before freezing batch-cooked meals, let them cool down entirely. Quick chilling keeps the food's quality intact and helps stop bacterial development. To expedite the chilling process, place containers in the refrigerator for a few hours or use an ice bath.

Meal Portioning: Before freezing, divide prepared meals into portions suitable for one person or a family. This keeps you from thawing more food than you need and makes it simple to get precisely what you need. For portioning out soups and sauces, think about using ice cube trays or silicone muffin cups.

Soups and sauces may be stored in freezer bags. Transfer liquids, such as soups and sauces, into freezer bags to save on storage space. To freeze the bags in a thin, even layer, place them flat on a baking sheet. To conserve freezer space, stack the bags vertically after they've frozen.

Freeze Ingredients Separately: If you want to utilize an ingredient in more than one recipe, freeze it separately. Freeze cooked grains, beans, and proteins separately, for instance, so you can combine them later to make different meals. This gives you more freedom to customize and vary your meals.

Rotate Your Freezer Stock: To make sure you consume the goods in your freezer before they go bad, rotate it regularly. Make a list of everything you have in your freezer, and use the oldest stuff first. To reduce food waste, think about putting in place a first-in, first-out (FIFO) system.

Properly Thaw Before Reheating: When frozen meals are ready to consume, thaw them overnight in the refrigerator or your microwave using the defrost option. Food should not be thawed at room temperature since this promotes the development of germs. Meals should be fully reheated to an internal temperature of 165°F (74°C) after they have thawed.

Type A dieters can save time and work in the kitchen while still enjoying tasty and nourishing meals that promote their health and well-being by adhering to these batch cooking and freezing techniques. Batch cooking and freezing may be effective strategies for maintaining a healthy diet and way of life with a little forethought and preparation.

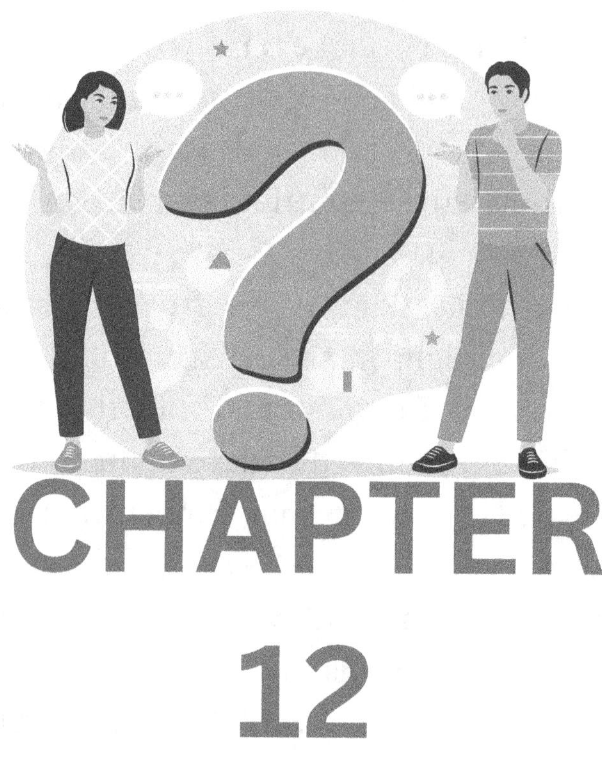

CHAPTER

12

Frequently Asked Questions (FAQs)

1.What is the Type A blood type diet?

·The Type A blood type diet is a nutritional approach that suggests individuals with Type A blood may benefit from eating certain foods while avoiding others based on their blood type.

2.How does the Type A blood type diet work?

·The Type A blood type diet is based on the premise that different blood types evolved at different times in history and may have adapted to different dietary patterns. It suggests that individuals with Type A blood may thrive on a primarily plant-based diet with limited amounts of animal protein.

3.What foods are recommended for Type A blood type?

·Foods recommended for Type A blood type typically include fresh fruits and vegetables, legumes, whole grains, tofu, seafood, and certain types of dairy. These foods are believed to support the digestive system and overall health of individuals with Type A blood.

4.What foods should be avoided on the Type A blood type diet?

·Foods that are typically avoided on the Type A blood type diet include red meat, processed meats, dairy products, certain types of grains, and some high-fat foods. These foods are believed to be less compatible with the digestive system of individuals with Type A blood.

5.Is there scientific evidence supporting the Type A blood type diet?

·While some proponents of the Type A blood type diet cite anecdotal evidence and personal testimonials, scientific research supporting its effectiveness is limited. More studies are needed to determine the validity and potential health benefits of this dietary approach.

6.Can the Type A blood type diet help with weight loss?

·Some individuals may experience weight loss on the Type A blood type diet due to its emphasis on whole, nutrient-dense foods and the avoidance of processed and high-fat foods. However, weight loss results can vary depending on individual factors such as metabolism, activity level, and overall diet quality.

7.Is the Type A blood type diet suitable for everyone with Type A blood?

·The Type A blood type diet is not a one-size-fits-all approach, and individual responses to dietary changes can vary. While some individuals with Type A blood may benefit from following this diet, others may not experience significant improvements in health or well-being.

8.Can I follow the Type A blood type diet if I have certain dietary restrictions or allergies?

·Individuals with dietary restrictions or allergies should consult with a healthcare professional before starting any new diet, including the Type A blood type diet. Modifications and substitutions may be necessary to accommodate specific dietary needs while still following the principles of the diet.

9.Are there any risks associated with the Type A blood type diet?

·While the Type A blood type diet emphasizes whole, nutritious foods, it may restrict certain food groups and nutrients, potentially leading to nutritional deficiencies if not properly balanced. It's important to ensure that all essential nutrients are obtained through dietary sources or supplementation.

10.Where can I find more information about the Type A blood type diet?
·Additional information about the Type A blood type diet can be found in books, online resources, and through consultation with healthcare professionals knowledgeable about nutrition and dietary interventions. It's essential to gather information from reputable sources and consider individual health needs and goals when exploring dietary approaches.

Conclusion

Finally, "Eat Well 4 Your Blood Type: A Customized Cookbook" offers a comprehensive dietary plan designed especially for those with Type A blood. We have discussed the idea of a blood-type-based diet throughout this cookbook, along with some possible advantages for general health and well-being.

Accepting the concepts of individualized nutrition, readers have found a plethora of healthy recipes that are carefully designed to meet the nutritional requirements of Type A personalities. Every meal, from breakfasts to desserts, has been carefully crafted to provide a harmonious combination of nutrients and scrumptious flavors.

We have examined the history, evolution, and scientific basis of blood-type diets, providing an in-depth look at this novel dietary strategy. After learning about the distinct qualities of Type A blood and its particular advantages, readers have learned important knowledge on how to best support their digestive health, control their weight, and maintain overall vigor via dietary choices.

Additionally, this cookbook offers helpful advice on how to confidently manage the kitchen, including suggestions for meal planning, quantity cooking, modification, and substitutes. We have encouraged readers to be flexible and creative in the kitchen by giving them the tools to make educated decisions and modify recipes to fit their preferences and lifestyles.

Let's take a trip of self-discovery and nourishment as we say goodbye to these pages. We'll embrace the ideas of tailored nutrition and enjoy the delectable tastes of healthful, Type A-friendly food. I hope that this cookbook becomes a reliable guide for you as you travel the road to bright health and well-being, leading you to a future full of vigor, happiness, and delicious food.

WEEKLY MEAL PLANNING

Month: ________________

Week: ① ② ③ ④

Sunday

Breakfast: ________________

Calories	Protein	Sugar	Carbs

Lunch: ________________

Calories	Protein	Sugar	Carbs

Dinner: ________________

Calories	Protein	Sugar	Carbs

Monday

Breakfast: ________________

Calories	Protein	Sugar	Carbs

Lunch: ________________

Calories	Protein	Sugar	Carbs

Dinner: ________________

Calories	Protein	Sugar	Carbs

Tuesday

Breakfast: ________________

Calories	Protein	Sugar	Carbs

Lunch: ________________

Calories	Protein	Sugar	Carbs

Dinner: ________________

Calories	Protein	Sugar	Carbs

Wednesday

Breakfast: ________________

Calories	Protein	Sugar	Carbs

Lunch: ________________

Calories	Protein	Sugar	Carbs

Dinner: ________________

Calories	Protein	Sugar	Carbs

Thursday

Breakfast: ________________

Calories	Protein	Sugar	Carbs

Lunch: ________________

Calories	Protein	Sugar	Carbs

Dinner: ________________

Calories	Protein	Sugar	Carbs

Friday

Breakfast: ________________

Calories	Protein	Sugar	Carbs

Lunch: ________________

Calories	Protein	Sugar	Carbs

Dinner: ________________

Calories	Protein	Sugar	Carbs

Saturday

Breakfast: ________________

Calories	Protein	Sugar	Carbs

Lunch: ________________

Calories	Protein	Sugar	Carbs

Dinner: ________________

Calories	Protein	Sugar	Carbs

Shopping List:

WEEKLY MEAL PLANNING

Month: _________________________

Week:

(1) (2) (3) (4)

Sunday

Breakfast: _______________

Calories	Protein	Sugar	Carbs

Lunch: _______________

Calories	Protein	Sugar	Carbs

Dinner: _______________

Calories	Protein	Sugar	Carbs

Monday

Breakfast: _______________

Calories	Protein	Sugar	Carbs

Lunch: _______________

Calories	Protein	Sugar	Carbs

Dinner: _______________

Calories	Protein	Sugar	Carbs

Tuesday

Breakfast: _______________

Calories	Protein	Sugar	Carbs

Lunch: _______________

Calories	Protein	Sugar	Carbs

Dinner: _______________

Calories	Protein	Sugar	Carbs

Wednesday

Breakfast: _______________

Calories	Protein	Sugar	Carbs

Lunch: _______________

Calories	Protein	Sugar	Carbs

Dinner: _______________

Calories	Protein	Sugar	Carbs

Thursday

Breakfast: _______________

Calories	Protein	Sugar	Carbs

Lunch: _______________

Calories	Protein	Sugar	Carbs

Dinner: _______________

Calories	Protein	Sugar	Carbs

Friday

Breakfast: _______________

Calories	Protein	Sugar	Carbs

Lunch: _______________

Calories	Protein	Sugar	Carbs

Dinner: _______________

Calories	Protein	Sugar	Carbs

Saturday

Breakfast: _______________

Calories	Protein	Sugar	Carbs

Lunch: _______________

Calories	Protein	Sugar	Carbs

Dinner: _______________

Calories	Protein	Sugar	Carbs

Shopping List:

WEEKLY MEAL PLANNING

Month: ______________________

Week:

(1) (2) (3) (4)

Sunday

Breakfast: ______________________

Calories	Protein	Sugar	Carbs

Lunch: ______________________

Calories	Protein	Sugar	Carbs

Dinner: ______________________

Calories	Protein	Sugar	Carbs

Monday

Breakfast: ______________________

Calories	Protein	Sugar	Carbs

Lunch: ______________________

Calories	Protein	Sugar	Carbs

Dinner: ______________________

Calories	Protein	Sugar	Carbs

Tuesday

Breakfast: ______________________

Calories	Protein	Sugar	Carbs

Lunch: ______________________

Calories	Protein	Sugar	Carbs

Dinner: ______________________

Calories	Protein	Sugar	Carbs

Wednesday

Breakfast: ______________________

Calories	Protein	Sugar	Carbs

Lunch: ______________________

Calories	Protein	Sugar	Carbs

Dinner: ______________________

Calories	Protein	Sugar	Carbs

Thursday

Breakfast: ______________________

Calories	Protein	Sugar	Carbs

Lunch: ______________________

Calories	Protein	Sugar	Carbs

Dinner: ______________________

Calories	Protein	Sugar	Carbs

Friday

Breakfast: ______________________

Calories	Protein	Sugar	Carbs

Lunch: ______________________

Calories	Protein	Sugar	Carbs

Dinner: ______________________

Calories	Protein	Sugar	Carbs

Saturday

Breakfast: ______________________

Calories	Protein	Sugar	Carbs

Lunch: ______________________

Calories	Protein	Sugar	Carbs

Dinner: ______________________

Calories	Protein	Sugar	Carbs

Shopping List:

WEEKLY MEAL PLANNING

Month: ______________________

Week:

(1) (2) (3) (4)

Sunday

Breakfast: ______________________

Calories	Protein	Sugar	Carbs

Lunch: ______________________

Calories	Protein	Sugar	Carbs

Dinner: ______________________

Calories	Protein	Sugar	Carbs

Monday

Breakfast: ______________________

Calories	Protein	Sugar	Carbs

Lunch: ______________________

Calories	Protein	Sugar	Carbs

Dinner: ______________________

Calories	Protein	Sugar	Carbs

Tuesday

Breakfast: ______________________

Calories	Protein	Sugar	Carbs

Lunch: ______________________

Calories	Protein	Sugar	Carbs

Dinner: ______________________

Calories	Protein	Sugar	Carbs

Wednesday

Breakfast: ______________________

Calories	Protein	Sugar	Carbs

Lunch: ______________________

Calories	Protein	Sugar	Carbs

Dinner: ______________________

Calories	Protein	Sugar	Carbs

Thursday

Breakfast: ______________________

Calories	Protein	Sugar	Carbs

Lunch: ______________________

Calories	Protein	Sugar	Carbs

Dinner: ______________________

Calories	Protein	Sugar	Carbs

Friday

Breakfast: ______________________

Calories	Protein	Sugar	Carbs

Lunch: ______________________

Calories	Protein	Sugar	Carbs

Dinner: ______________________

Calories	Protein	Sugar	Carbs

Saturday

Breakfast: ______________________

Calories	Protein	Sugar	Carbs

Lunch: ______________________

Calories	Protein	Sugar	Carbs

Dinner: ______________________

Calories	Protein	Sugar	Carbs

Shopping List:

WEEKLY MEAL PLANNING

Month: ______________________

Week:

(1) (2) (3) (4)

Sunday

Breakfast: ______________________

Calories	Protein	Sugar	Carbs

Lunch: ______________________

Calories	Protein	Sugar	Carbs

Dinner: ______________________

Calories	Protein	Sugar	Carbs

Monday

Breakfast: ______________________

Calories	Protein	Sugar	Carbs

Lunch: ______________________

Calories	Protein	Sugar	Carbs

Dinner: ______________________

Calories	Protein	Sugar	Carbs

Tuesday

Breakfast: ______________________

Calories	Protein	Sugar	Carbs

Lunch: ______________________

Calories	Protein	Sugar	Carbs

Dinner: ______________________

Calories	Protein	Sugar	Carbs

Wednesday

Breakfast: ______________________

Calories	Protein	Sugar	Carbs

Lunch: ______________________

Calories	Protein	Sugar	Carbs

Dinner: ______________________

Calories	Protein	Sugar	Carbs

Thursday

Breakfast: ______________________

Calories	Protein	Sugar	Carbs

Lunch: ______________________

Calories	Protein	Sugar	Carbs

Dinner: ______________________

Calories	Protein	Sugar	Carbs

Friday

Breakfast: ______________________

Calories	Protein	Sugar	Carbs

Lunch: ______________________

Calories	Protein	Sugar	Carbs

Dinner: ______________________

Calories	Protein	Sugar	Carbs

Saturday

Breakfast: ______________________

Calories	Protein	Sugar	Carbs

Lunch: ______________________

Calories	Protein	Sugar	Carbs

Dinner: ______________________

Calories	Protein	Sugar	Carbs

Shopping List:

WEEKLY MEAL PLANNING

Month: _______________

Week:

(1) (2) (3) (4)

Sunday

Breakfast: _______________

Calories	Protein	Sugar	Carbs

Lunch: _______________

Calories	Protein	Sugar	Carbs

Dinner: _______________

Calories	Protein	Sugar	Carbs

Monday

Breakfast: _______________

Calories	Protein	Sugar	Carbs

Lunch: _______________

Calories	Protein	Sugar	Carbs

Dinner: _______________

Calories	Protein	Sugar	Carbs

Tuesday

Breakfast: _______________

Calories	Protein	Sugar	Carbs

Lunch: _______________

Calories	Protein	Sugar	Carbs

Dinner: _______________

Calories	Protein	Sugar	Carbs

Wednesday

Breakfast: _______________

Calories	Protein	Sugar	Carbs

Lunch: _______________

Calories	Protein	Sugar	Carbs

Dinner: _______________

Calories	Protein	Sugar	Carbs

Thursday

Breakfast: _______________

Calories	Protein	Sugar	Carbs

Lunch: _______________

Calories	Protein	Sugar	Carbs

Dinner: _______________

Calories	Protein	Sugar	Carbs

Friday

Breakfast: _______________

Calories	Protein	Sugar	Carbs

Lunch: _______________

Calories	Protein	Sugar	Carbs

Dinner: _______________

Calories	Protein	Sugar	Carbs

Saturday

Breakfast: _______________

Calories	Protein	Sugar	Carbs

Lunch: _______________

Calories	Protein	Sugar	Carbs

Dinner: _______________

Calories	Protein	Sugar	Carbs

Shopping List:

WEEKLY MEAL PLANNING

Month: ______________________

Week:

(1) (2) (3) (4)

Sunday

Breakfast: ______________________

Calories	Protein	Sugar	Carbs

Lunch: ______________________

Calories	Protein	Sugar	Carbs

Dinner: ______________________

Calories	Protein	Sugar	Carbs

Monday

Breakfast: ______________________

Calories	Protein	Sugar	Carbs

Lunch: ______________________

Calories	Protein	Sugar	Carbs

Dinner: ______________________

Calories	Protein	Sugar	Carbs

Tuesday

Breakfast: ______________________

Calories	Protein	Sugar	Carbs

Lunch: ______________________

Calories	Protein	Sugar	Carbs

Dinner: ______________________

Calories	Protein	Sugar	Carbs

Wednesday

Breakfast: ______________________

Calories	Protein	Sugar	Carbs

Lunch: ______________________

Calories	Protein	Sugar	Carbs

Dinner: ______________________

Calories	Protein	Sugar	Carbs

Thursday

Breakfast: ______________________

Calories	Protein	Sugar	Carbs

Lunch: ______________________

Calories	Protein	Sugar	Carbs

Dinner: ______________________

Calories	Protein	Sugar	Carbs

Friday

Breakfast: ______________________

Calories	Protein	Sugar	Carbs

Lunch: ______________________

Calories	Protein	Sugar	Carbs

Dinner: ______________________

Calories	Protein	Sugar	Carbs

Saturday

Breakfast: ______________________

Calories	Protein	Sugar	Carbs

Lunch: ______________________

Calories	Protein	Sugar	Carbs

Dinner: ______________________

Calories	Protein	Sugar	Carbs

Shopping List:

WEEKLY MEAL PLANNING

Month: ____________________

Week:

(1) (2) (3) (4)

Sunday

Breakfast: ____________________

Calories	Protein	Sugar	Carbs

Lunch: ____________________

Calories	Protein	Sugar	Carbs

Dinner: ____________________

Calories	Protein	Sugar	Carbs

Monday

Breakfast: ____________________

Calories	Protein	Sugar	Carbs

Lunch: ____________________

Calories	Protein	Sugar	Carbs

Dinner: ____________________

Calories	Protein	Sugar	Carbs

Tuesday

Breakfast: ____________________

Calories	Protein	Sugar	Carbs

Lunch: ____________________

Calories	Protein	Sugar	Carbs

Dinner: ____________________

Calories	Protein	Sugar	Carbs

Wednesday

Breakfast: ____________________

Calories	Protein	Sugar	Carbs

Lunch: ____________________

Calories	Protein	Sugar	Carbs

Dinner: ____________________

Calories	Protein	Sugar	Carbs

Thursday

Breakfast: ____________________

Calories	Protein	Sugar	Carbs

Lunch: ____________________

Calories	Protein	Sugar	Carbs

Dinner: ____________________

Calories	Protein	Sugar	Carbs

Friday

Breakfast: ____________________

Calories	Protein	Sugar	Carbs

Lunch: ____________________

Calories	Protein	Sugar	Carbs

Dinner: ____________________

Calories	Protein	Sugar	Carbs

Saturday

Breakfast: ____________________

Calories	Protein	Sugar	Carbs

Lunch: ____________________

Calories	Protein	Sugar	Carbs

Dinner: ____________________

Calories	Protein	Sugar	Carbs

Shopping List:

WEEKLY MEAL PLANNING

Month: ____________________

Week: (1) (2) (3) (4)

Sunday

Breakfast: ____________________

Calories	Protein	Sugar	Carbs

Lunch: ____________________

Calories	Protein	Sugar	Carbs

Dinner: ____________________

Calories	Protein	Sugar	Carbs

Monday

Breakfast: ____________________

Calories	Protein	Sugar	Carbs

Lunch: ____________________

Calories	Protein	Sugar	Carbs

Dinner: ____________________

Calories	Protein	Sugar	Carbs

Tuesday

Breakfast: ____________________

Calories	Protein	Sugar	Carbs

Lunch: ____________________

Calories	Protein	Sugar	Carbs

Dinner: ____________________

Calories	Protein	Sugar	Carbs

Wednesday

Breakfast: ____________________

Calories	Protein	Sugar	Carbs

Lunch: ____________________

Calories	Protein	Sugar	Carbs

Dinner: ____________________

Calories	Protein	Sugar	Carbs

Thursday

Breakfast: ____________________

Calories	Protein	Sugar	Carbs

Lunch: ____________________

Calories	Protein	Sugar	Carbs

Dinner: ____________________

Calories	Protein	Sugar	Carbs

Friday

Breakfast: ____________________

Calories	Protein	Sugar	Carbs

Lunch: ____________________

Calories	Protein	Sugar	Carbs

Dinner: ____________________

Calories	Protein	Sugar	Carbs

Saturday

Breakfast: ____________________

Calories	Protein	Sugar	Carbs

Lunch: ____________________

Calories	Protein	Sugar	Carbs

Dinner: ____________________

Calories	Protein	Sugar	Carbs

Shopping List: